HEALTHCARE PROVIDERS
ULITMATE GUIDE
TO WIN
Even As Medicare
Changes the Rules

Mark Kimmel, Ph.D.

HEALTHCARE PROVIDERS

ULTIMATE GUIDE TO WIN

EVEN AS MEDICARE CHANGES THE RULES

Mark Kimmel, Ph.D.

TOPLINE Healthcare
Great Falls, VA 22066
www.toplinehealthcare.com

FIRST EDITION

Format and Layout by Hemco Publishing

Chief Editor: Susan Hemme

ISBN- 978-1492356714

This book is dedicated

to the memory of my Father,

the ever-present joy of my Mother, and

to every Healthcare Provider who stands in

the face of change and contributes

to making our world a better,

healthier place to live

.

CONTENTS

PREFACE

Hello and welcome to the new age of healthcare. My name is Mark Kimmel and I am here to help you thrive and come out ahead of the changes in Medicare (as the title says) even as Medicare changes the rules. I will tell you more about myself in Chapter 1, but for now, I'd like to tell you about this book and why I wrote it for you.

I have worked in the healthcare industry and with providers for over 20 years. I see how difficult it is for everyone to not only keep up with all of the changes, but also to understand why these changes are so important and how they directly affect you. This led me down a path to create a solution that directly helps you, as well as helps to create a culture of healthcare professionals who work together in alignment with Medicare.

So go ahead and get comfortable. This is an easy-read loaded with information that is vital for your awareness so you will know what to do and how to act before it's too late.

This book addresses a number of changes in areas of our industry such as how you are required to document, clinical validation, changing to ICD-10*, RAC* audits, the appeals process, reimbursement reversals, converting to electronic medical records, use of your NPI* number, and so on.

* Acronyms are defined in the following Chapters and in the Index in the back of the book.

These changes will have a massive impact on you as a provider, and if you are not aware of them now or don't know what to do, they will potentially cause you financial harm and make your life miserable. But don't worry; I will explain throughout this book what these changes are, what they mean to you, how you can protect and position yourself, and how you can be proactive to come out ahead of the game.

My purpose in writing this book is to give you a starting point to help you to build on your experiences, expand your knowledge, and understand where the healthcare industry is headed. I intend to strengthen you as a provider, and to do so in a way that helps you save time and money, and supports you so that you are freed up to give better quality care to your patients. Wouldn't this make your life better?

On a daily basis, I have worked with a diverse group of doctors. I see that they do the best they can to do the right thing. They work hard and are consistently being pushed to document more and to be more specific. Those doctors constantly asked, "WHY am I having to do this when I give good care?" I figured if they are asking why, then others in the industry must be asking the same question. As it turns out, you are. And so are your colleagues.

Providers need help, and I want to help them. So I went on a quest to become expertly informed and to see what I could do. I found a great deal of information from a volume of sources that most providers never knew about. Then, I started taking classes, sitting for exams and getting certified in skills that directly helped me to help you.

I am passionate to learn, expand and grow. And with the subject being Medicare, you can never stop learning as it is always growing and changing. Just as you think you have it mastered, new changes appear. Then a new adventure begins all over again. The challenge is actually very exciting!

As I implemented what I learned, along with expanding my skills and working together as a team, the doctors I worked with experienced drastic improvement. Our numbers as a hospital went up, work flows improved and a phenomenal amount of money was saved. Let me assure you, if you are holding this book in your hands, then you have just taken your first step to experience the same.

I have designed this book to help you understand how everything is interconnected. At times it may seem repetitive, but stay with me. It is meant to help you learn why so much of your time is currently spent doing things such as writing your progress notes. I will teach you how this can be improved and what you can do to make your life as a physician more simplified. Knowing what Medicare expects and knowing what is behind what you are required to do empowers you to make the right decisions. This book will help you do this.

This book is not intended to be a done-for-you, read-it-and-forget-it-instant-solution to the problem. We're not dealing with a one-time problem that has an easy fix. It won't help you to just read this then put it aside and hope for the best. It is intended to be a done-with-you, let's-team-up-together-solution where I help you obtain information you need to know so that you can begin shifting now and get ahead of the changes that are coming as well as changes that are already in effect.

As you can see, I had you as the provider in mind as I wrote this book. I have reached out to hundreds of our colleagues and listened to their opinions, questions, fears and concerns. I have discovered that there is a tremendous urgency and need in our industry to understand what is going on with the changes in Medicare's Rules and Regulations.

Having this information is vital to every healthcare provider in the nation. This is what motivates me to forge ahead and keeps our team building in strength in order to bring the right information, systems and tools to you.

I am very humble to be in a place to offer you this book. This entire process has been amazing, from writing the book to co-founding Topline Healthcare, a company that brings you solutions to the Medicare problem. I will admit it has not been easy. But, I'm sure that as a physician, you can relate to what it's like to relentlessly push yourself in order to truly make a difference. Call me crazy, but this is what I do.

I am most fortunate to have the tremendous support of people around me who are on the same page. I'd like to acknowledge all of the people I have worked with, especially the wonderful group of doctors for their valuable input, James Rodgers, MD., for his unwavering support, and Hayley Bieker for sharing her vast knowledge of coding and documentation.

I thank my Topline Healthcare business partner and dear friend, Susan Hemme for keeping me on the right path and for her endless support in helping me to make things happen.

And I give special appreciation to all of you reading this book. I appreciate you for taking the time to hear what I have to say. I know your lives are extremely busy and I want you to know that I don't take that lightly.

Know that I am here to serve you with limitless gratitude and absolute dedication to your success.

Chapter 1

Playing to Win

You don't have to listen to me. I'm just a nerd. However, everybody needs a nerd. My guess is you are refined and highly skilled at what you do. I bet you can multi-task, multi-think and multi-achieve anything you want on many levels. You went into this medical profession because you enjoy helping people and solving problems. You're good at what you do, and there's not much that you can't handle.

Then why is it you are reading a book like this? Is it Medicare? Is it because you are concerned about the changes that have a grip on this country? Do you want to better understand what these changes are? Do you want to know what else is coming down the pipe? Are you uncertain as to how all of this will affect you? Your career? Your family? Your lifestyle?

Well, let me tell you, you're in the right place and you are not alone.

Ever since Medicare changed the rules and created this giant arm of claw backs, perfectly good healthcare providers, just like you, are standing like bowling pins in the line of a big, heavy ball that's ready to strike. It is perfectly understandable to be concerned about how this might throw you and/or your hospital in the gutter.

No worries. With the right team in place, you can accomplish anything, and this is where I come in. We team up.

Because of my current confidentiality agreement, I cannot state the actual dollar amount, but I can tell you that I have consistently saved my hospital an exorbitant amount of money with a program for documentation that meets the Centers for Medicare & Medicaid Services (CMS) and Medicare guidelines while aligning you with the changes that are coming. I have created a system that keeps us ahead of the game so that when you document, you have everything required of you in one component. You are then speaking in what I have coined, 'Codeable Language', which not only applies to the bill, but also puts you at an advantage for your future and how you are publically ranked as a physician. Not bad for a nerd, right? Okay then, maybe you should listen to me.

WHO IS HURT AND HOW CAN I HELP?

I know what it's like to fight for something when you have no choice but to win. On September 14, 1999, I was faced with this challenge while working in the ICU at a hospital in Orange County, California. The morning started out pretty much like any other day with the hospital taking in patients, tending to their needs, prepping for surgery, etc. I was on call for code duty, but uneventfully going about my business and routinely taking vital signs of a gentleman who had come in following a heart attack.

Suddenly, shots rang out! A disgruntled gunman unmercifully attacked, killing three of my fellow employees: a nurse, the director of pharmacy and the maintenance supervisor. Code Gray turned into Code Blue as the ripple effect spread and reality took hold of the hospital. This was not a drill. My mind went into overdrive thinking, "Who is hurt and how can I help?"

I ran towards the screams as terrified patients were diving for cover, however my efforts were blocked as I was turned back by more gunfire. Fortunately, police then apprehended the gunman. Unfortunately, it was not until after he had shot his third victim, as a young mother in the lobby while she was protecting her two young children.

This incident affected life on so many levels. Innocent people were killed. Bystanders were terrorized. The lives of families, forever changed. Our place of work no longer felt healthy or safe. There seemed to be no sense as to why this had happened. So many thoughts ran through my mind following that event. My life was severely impacted. I wanted to shut down and leave, perhaps go somewhere else and start over. However I knew that if I did, not only would I be letting this monster win, but I also would be letting down the very people that I am committed to help and serve.

It was important for me to fight for my life and win the battle within myself following that horrific incident. I reached deep within to find the cause as well as find a solution for moving forward. Then, with the help of family, friends, and amazing heroes like you, we teamed up and together we won.

Although a hospital shooting is not exactly what you are dealing with as a provider, there is still that sense of being a target of sudden change that is out of your control. Having everything you do affected by someone else's decision can make you feel like you are in a loosing position, like you have nowhere to turn. I am here, alive and well, to tell you that with a committed nerd like me on your side and with what I have to share, you are certainly not alone. You can and will come out ahead, even as Medicare changes the rules.

FIGHT FOR YOUR RIGHT

So what are some of those changes? On January 1, 2010 it became required by law that the Recovery Audit Contractor (RAC) program, was to be in effect and reinforced in every state in America. Unfortunately, like those shots fired in my hospital in 1999, this act is causing a ripple effect of reaction that is changing the face of healthcare, as we know it, throughout our nation.

The mission of RAC is to review, audit, identify and take back what they deem to be improper Medicare payments to you. They are set up to reduce fraud, improve healthcare and help reduce the federal deficit.

Fair enough, right? No. Because being the government, Medicare can arbitrarily change the playing field in order to slant the rules in their favor. They can do this by requiring you speak to them in a language that only they know, and then leave it to you to find out what that language is. We may be on the same page as far as reducing fraud, improving healthcare and helping to reduce the federal deficit. However, we're not on the same page if this means throwing you and your career under the bus. There is another way.

I fought for my life and for those I cared about. Now I am

fighting for you. The win is easy since we are using Medicare's own language, own rules and own regulations to give them what they want while accomplishing what we need as providers. I know this works because I've already proven it.

THE PROOF'S IN THE PUDDING

At one of our nation's top hospitals where I have worked in Southern California, I assisted the Adult Hospitalist program with quality improvement in care and documentation. With my understanding of technology and computers, I was able to use what we had, in terms of a highbred electronic system in combination with educational solutions, to improve our billing and Hierarchical Condition Categories (HCC) scores. Our coding compliance scores soared from 65% to 93% across the board, in less than a year. By leaning out the process and applying my Codeable Language™ system, I helped the hospital to save time, make things work more efficiently, reduce litigation and increase reimbursements from Medicare. Pretty cool, huh?

I am known as the "computer nerd" having worked on a build for several parts of the computer systems we used (from the computerized progress note with Medicare language built in, to the billing component built into the note) so that the billing is done when your note is completed. Since I have been both an advisor to physicians as well as a nurse, I see things from both sides of the coin. Truly understanding how physicians work gives me an advantage in building systems and designing programs. Knowing what is important to you as well as knowing the administrative end is what helps bridge the divide between profitability and quality of care.

As the Clinical Care Coordinator of the Adult Hospitalists, I was able to see the broader picture from multi-points of view. I was an extension of the Medical Director of Health Plans and the Independent Practice Association (IPA). I was the Clinical Care Manager for Hospitalist Services, in charge of the hospitalist and their documentation and compliance. This position was a multi-faceted role where I worked as a liaison between the health plans and the hospital. I am experienced in case management, payroll and HR issues, just to name a few...

(Okay, my editor put all of this in here so you would know the strengths of who is going to bat for you on your team. So here's more...)

Professionally, being a Certified RAC Coordinator, a Certified Clinical Documentation Improvement Specialist and a Certified Lean Trainer, not only am I known as the nerd, I am known for leadership, clinical knowledge and complex understanding of work flows. I am very linear in thought in order to make sure that what we do and how it is done is a thriving process that it is quickly replicable and cost reducing. Basically, I do what is takes to make things work.

I MAKE THINGS WORK

I make things work so that you are strategically positioned to win in this game where physician documentation is headed. You will see this more clearly in the following chapters where I discuss what's here and now, what's trending for the future and how all of this is going to affect you. I will walk you through the changes with Medicare and RAC audits and what all this means to your reimbursements.

We will go into the electronic expectations, consequences of non-compliance, and what you can start doing now to protect yourself from unnecessary penalties. I will also provide you with solutions to help you with the technological side of medicine, which is changing at unprecedented speed.

Understanding the Thread of this Book

Throughout this book you may notice the same subject mentioned in several different ways. I have done this in an effort to show you how interconnected this process is and how important your understanding of it is today. I have used the same illustration so that you can see the many layers needed in your documentation to ensure your success. Each part of this process is important to understand. How it works together may seem repetitive, yet be assured, it is only used to paint the clear picture needed for proper payment from the hard work you do.

Shall we get started?

Mark Kimmel, Ph.D.

Chapter 2

Medicare's Tidal Wave of Change

Change is here. You can see it. You can feel it. You know it. Everybody's talking about it. And if you are like most healthcare providers, then you too are facing an uphill battle with reimbursement. You are doing the work. You are providing good care. Yet when it comes to documentation and the way Medicare is radically changing, you are not being fully compensated for the work you do or valued as the quality care provider that you are.

While the intention of the Affordable Care Act of 2012 may be to provide "Quality Affordable Health Care for all Americans," we all know that it is making things more difficult for you as a provider to administer that quality care. Therefore, the purpose of this book is to give you insight into how the recent changes directly affect you and what you can do to win. When you have the right information and tools, and know what to do with it, you are able to do what you do best. And that is to provide quality healthcare.

With our ever-changing healthcare system, there are key points necessary for you to thrive as a healthcare provider.

You must first understand the players of the game, the rules that are changing, how you must adapt to meet those new rules and regulations and what kind of team and defense you need to build in order to get ahead and stay ahead. As you know, the rules and regulations are rapidly changing. So what I will be providing are the more important rules that you need to know along with what you must do. Along with this, I strongly advise you to continually seek education and actively search for more specifics. The more you know, the better you are positioned to stay ahead of the game.

NEW RULES, NEW GAME

This is a key point: In the next three to ten years the Baby Boomers will hit as the largest number of enrollees in Medicare history. Foreseeing this, the government is tightening up their purse strings now. They are making a major shift in cost savings in an effort to keep the system running. One of the most effective ways for them to do this is to make new rules and change the game in their favor. They will do this because they can; they are the government.

The intended outcome may be to improve efficiency in the healthcare system, however changes such as switching from ICD-9 to ICD-10 (International Statistical Classifications of Diseases current codes in use), greater focus on clinical validation and RAC audits puts the burden of compliance, time, energy and cost on you.

The Centers for Medicare and Medicaid Services (CMS) will be taking aggressive strides to accelerate the acceptance of evidence-based healthcare and collect on perceived overpayments to providers to help lighten the load of a strained national budget. After spending the past 30 years collecting and analyzing outcomes data from internal programs such as Comprehensive Error Rate Testing (CERT), Hospital Payment Monitoring Program (HPMP), and Quality Improvement Organization (QIOs), both Congress and CMS have committed unprecedented resources to enforce evidence-based coverage policies and stop what they perceive to be Medicare fraud.

This is Important:
Medicare is the gold standard in the entire country when it comes to billing.

So when Medicare implements a rule, every health plan follows to some degree. Even if you do not accept Medicare, most health plans will follow the guidelines set forth by Medicare. You and every provider that documents in order to provide billing to a health plan, must follow the Medicare guidelines.

However, what you may not be fully aware of is how these guidelines are changing and how those changes affect you. Not only is it important how you document in order to get paid, but also how you are ultimately perceived as a physician in the public eye.

There are many areas where Medicare has increased rules and regulations that directly affect how you document and how you get paid. The most important areas that you need to pay close attention to are: (1) Changing from ICD-9 to ICD-10, (2) Clinical Validation, (3) RAC Audits, (4) the high cost of appeals, (5) mandate for electronic medical records and (6) the ranking system that will be linked to your NPI number.

CHANGING TO ICD-10

As a better method in detecting Medicare fraud, changing from ICD-9 to ICD-10 is intended to make the billing process more efficient while providing greater precision in data. However, making the switch to ICD-10 is both costly and time-intensive. It requires business, clinical and system changes throughout your organization. Practice management software and payment policies need to be updated. Also, as documentation requirements change, communication between providers and coders becomes more important than ever before.

You will need to provide solid documentation that supports the increased details of ICD-10. You must start *now* to minimize the effects of these changes on your reimbursement. You need to understand what Medicare is looking for. It is to your benefit to recognize that Medicare is a government-based program, and every government-based program has a numbering system. That numbering system for you is the Diagnosis Related Group (DRG), but do you know whether it is attached to an ICD-9 or an ICD-10?

Medicare is not only requiring you to understand which code belongs to which diagnosis, they are now asking you to be more specific in everything you write. The problem is that even with all the education sent out by CMS, providers do not have the time to read all of the information to document correctly. And if you don't submit it in their required language, then they don't have to pay you.

For Example

Although you may know what category in which to place pneumonia, do you have the correct code for pneumonia? Is this a community-acquired pneumonia? Is this a facility-acquired pneumonia? Is this pneumonia caused streptococcus? The type of pneumonia is now going to need specification as well as its location... left lung...right lung...bilateral? Whereas before, a physician could write pneumonia and you were done. Now your documentation has to give the right codes as well as completely tell the full story of your patient.

How you document now, how you treat your patient and the outcomes are all tied together.

Under the new rules, you are going to be publically ranked according as to how well you document along with the outcomes of your patient – not one or the other. These are now holding equal weight. This means that you can be the best physician on the planet, properly caring for your patients, but if you don't properly document exactly what was done, you will become subject to audits and take backs as well as being ranked as a poor physician (more on this below and in Chapter 3).

Until now, knowing how to document was fairly straightforward. You could simply state the basics of what was going on with your patient, submit the bill, and get paid. Now, you must be prepared to use the proper required codes and wording to go along with those codes in order to get paid for the work you do.

Most providers have never been taught to do this. We have all learned to speak in the way of the medical community, however what you really need to know now is how to speak in a complete language that is coded and acceptable to Medicare, or you won't get paid.

Medicare's Language

Knowing how to document is only part of the fight. You must also be prepared to use the proper required wording in order to get paid for all of the work you do. You must speak in Medicare's accepted language using codes and words that are acceptable to them.

Why, you might ask? Because, Medicare is a government-based payment option. If you know anything about the government, not only does everything work on codes, but everything works according to their rules. If you want a No. 2 pencil, you have to know the right code for that particular No. 2 pencil, as well as having to describe that pencil in the words they want to hear. Otherwise, you won't get the pencil that you want. In other words, you have to know the code as well as the description, because you can have the right code and the wrong description, or visa versa, and your request will be denied.

The same thing applies to clinical documentation with validation. If you don't have the right codes with the right language behind those codes, Medicare does not have to pay you. Or they won't pay you in full. Subsequently, if you are paid and they later decide to audit you, then they can take your money back. Either way, they win. You must play their game by their rules. You have no choice.

CLINICAL VALIDATION

Clinical validation is the process of determining whether evidence in the medical records, such as signs and symptoms, diagnostic test results and treatments, supports the diagnosis code. However, now your documentation practically needs to read like a well-written biography of your patient. You need to tell the full story.

Previously when we would document, we could simply go in the chart, document a value such as potassium at 2.7, patient is stable, and we would be done. Today, you need to list that you have a sixty-four year old male who presented signs and symptoms of diastolic heart failure, CAD, type II diabetes, has been getting 40mg of Lasix times three, with a weight loss of four pounds, BMP of 3100, hypokalemia, as indicated by a potassium of 2.7, replace potassium per pharmacy protocol, will continue to monitor, will reevaluate with CBC, CXR and Lasix 40mg in the am.

As you can see, this is a dramatic change to the current practice for most providers. This is intended to not only reduce fraud, but also to create a consistent and clear language that all providers understand. This also reinforces clinical validation.

In an effort to reduce claim denials, coders query physicians for more information. However, clinical validation makes it more difficult. Medicare auditors are denying claims that can't be clinically validated in the medical records, even if the code matches the diagnosis. Therefore, prior to code assignment, the coder will issue a query to you in order to get clarification when there is conflicting, incomplete, or ambiguous information in the health record.

It's important for you to remember is that the admitting physician is the one submitting the claim. This is why your interpretation of the clinical information is key to the success of reimbursement. Medicare states that you are the one to make all final determinations. This means that even if you have one of the world's premier specialists assisting you on this case, your documentations are the only ones that Medicare will consider. Therefore, it is important that you read and understand what your consultants have stated.

For Example

Your patient comes to the ER and the ER physicians say to rule out CHF, rule out MI, and rule out GERD. Your Cardiologist states positive Non-Stemi. You, as the attending provider, must address what has been stated. Medicare cannot take the word of the Cardiologist. You must put in your documentation a "Non-Stemi, no CHF or GERD noted". Yes, that is correct. You, as the attending physician, are required to make the final diagnosis.

Coders are Not Clinicians

The problem is, as you take care of your patients and document the best you can, you hand off your notes to coders, who typically are not clinicians. They sit behind a program, take what you've written, and enter the data while their brains are attempting to figure out what it is you are trying to say. If they don't understand what you are trying to say, you then get queried. They send you a sheet asking all sorts of questions. You will now have to go back into the medical records, review what was done, and try to figure out what the coder is asking of you.

Have you ever noticed that when your coder queries you, they tend to ask you indirect questions? That's because the job of coders is bound by rules and regulations. And though they require knowledge of medical terminology, coders are generally non-clinical personnel whose main duties are to analyze clinical statements and assign standardized codes using a classification system in order to write the bill.

In today's rules and regulations, Medicare says the coders cannot lead you or prompt you. Therefore, coders can only ask you indirect questions in order to determine what you are trying to say on your note.

For Example

They can ask you questions that can be answered yes, no or undetermined i.e., "Was this present on admission?"; "Was this pneumonia?". They cannot ask you if this is aspiration pneumonia or community acquired pneumonia with klebsiella.

Coders are not allowed to prompt you. They have to be a clinician in order for them to ask those types of questions. And coders are generally not clinicians. If you allow them to ask those types of direct questions, then you would have a case-of-leading, and that would lead you to the possibility of Medicare fraud.

You Are Ultimately Responsible

Coders can help in the effort to convert to ICD-10 by ensuring that you have access to checklists or other tools that summarize the documentation required for diagnosis. However, the burden of telling the full story of your patient falls on you. And if you don't tell the full story using the proper documentation, and you get audited, Medicare may also deem that to be fraud.

With that being said, giving you an opportunity to choose from a list of options would not be leading according to Medicare. We'll go into this further in Chapter 5 where I talk about the software, Codeable Language™, as a tool that helps you paint the full picture of your patient while making it easier on your coders and giving Medicare what they want.

Another point to consider is that coders generally are non-clinical, yet they are able to understand the diagnosis and what it means on the bill. This is because they use computer programs that help them follow a trend. They will read to you what you wrote as the reason for admission. As the admitting physician, you must determine the admitting diagnosis. The coder will then review your chart for certain key words that will lead them to believe that something is there. If they are uncertain, they will issue a query.

You will begin to see repetitive things that can lead you down a path to a medical judgment. As the provider, you are trained to make that decision. Here's the problem: if you lack supporting documentation for that path, according to Medicare, you are possibly committing fraud. This is why a coder cannot lead you. They may know that X equals Y, but they don't know that in order to get there you will need to have clinical signs, symptoms, tests and other items underneath to support it. They simply don't have the clinical component to be able to put the puzzle together and get the correct answer. That's your job.

Once your note gets past the coder, it is reviewed by finance, and then submitted for reimbursement. If the submission is not precisely written in a codeable language that is acceptable by Medicare, the claim is denied. Or worse, if the claim gets paid, and later with the new rules you are audited and your money gets taken back, your lifestyle could be greatly affected. Most likely you will have already spent that money on your mortgage, college tuition or an amazing trip to Antarctica. However, none of that matters to the government.

The Health Information Management (HIM) department within a hospital or organization is responsible for the legal care and appropriate distribution of medical records. They have been charged with sending out the bills through their coding department. However, Medicare now states that you as the provider, you and you alone, are ultimately responsible for what is on that bill. Although HIM is responsible for your bills and for your charts, Medicare is still targeting you, the physician.

As a result, you will be spending more time being concerned about what to write so that you don't get queried, or about the possibility of being targeted by Medicare. This means that instead of spending more time with your patients and practicing medicine, you will be spending more time documenting and needing to defend yourself. And it doesn't stop there.

RAC AUDITS

The Recovery Audit Contractor (RAC) program was created through the Medicare Modernization Act of 2003. Their purpose is to identify and recover improper Medicare payments paid to healthcare providers under fee-for-service Medicare plans. Then, under section 302 of the Tax Relief and Health Care Act of 2006, the United States Department of Health and Human Services (DHHS) was required by law to make the program permanent for all states by January 1, 2010. This caused a wave of RAC audits that is taking the nation by storm.

Hospitals Closing Down

Several hospitals throughout the United States are closing down today because of the Medicare RAC audits. In 2013, RAC took back $744.8 million dollars in the first quarter alone. They took back $2.29 billion (BILLION) in 2012, and $4.8 billion since 2010. They are taking back so much money that hospitals are losing capital and not able to keep their doors open.

Under the new rules, Medicare will be going after physicians as well. Not only are they penalizing the hospital, they are now positioning to penalize you.

Army of Auditors

In addition to the highly touted and widely publicized RAC audits, Medicare Zone Program Integrity Contractors (ZPIC) audits, Office of the Inspector General (OIG) audits, Department of Justice (DOJ) audits, Medicaid Integrity Contractor audits and the Medicare One PI system are just samples of the latest initiatives focused on provider payments.

However, Centers for Medicare and Medicaid Services (CMS) is adopting RAC audits as the first real tangible effort to push hospitals, physicians and other healthcare providers down a path of revolutionizing the clinical practice of medicine. CMS has combined clinical pay-for-performance (P4P) incentives and value-based purchasing initiatives with the strong arm of RAC medical collection agencies to insure providers are doing their part to facilitate a more nationalized, evidence-based healthcare structure.

In a nutshell, this means every hospital, every physician, and every healthcare provider in the United States will now be subject to the scrutiny of audits, claw backs and penalties. This is Medicare's offensive play to minimize reimbursements and maximize their ability to recoup perceived overpayments.

Reimbursement Reversals

According to CMS.gov, "Beginning in 2015, Medicare eligible professionals who do not successfully demonstrate meaningful use will be subject to a payment adjustment."

For years you have known that Medicare has gone after hospitals and institutions for reimbursement when the documentation did not support the care of the patients. Up until 2013, this has not affected you. However, they are now going to do the same thing to physicians that for years they have been doing to the hospitals. With the new changes, every physician today doing business, who accepts Medicare, is open for RAC audits and reimbursement reversal, which means Medicare can take your money back. Okay, now that you've got that, let's move on.

Audits and Claw Backs Affecting All Providers

Starting in the year 2015, hospitals, physicians and all healthcare providers will be required to document to a level never seen before in history; this is referring to anyone who documents to receive reimbursement from Medicare. Levels of care, lengths of stay, outcomes, overpayments and readmissions will all have new penalties that directly affect every provider that offers care in the United States. And Medicare Recovery Auditors are watching you now.

It is projected that by 2021 or so Medicare will be out of money if they continue to work as they currently do. As you know, with any business model with a projection of failure, steps must be taken to correct it. Medicare is finding that there's a lot of "waste, fraud and abuse" (in their opinion) within the system. Based upon these findings, they have changed the rules so that they can take money back.

For many years, hospitals have been fined or have had money taken back because they did not have the correct documentation or the physician didn't document something appropriately. And it wasn't until the last few years that taking money back from the physicians was even discussed. This is a basic case of where demand has outweighed the money that can be spent on patient care. We now need to look at new and innovative ways of making things work.

One way that Medicare has done this is by scrutinizing the bill to ensure accuracy. Another way will be with the new changes taking full effect in 2015. If Medicare deems that you did not document properly, they can go back as far as five years, perform an audit, and recoup money from you. Until now, you were somewhat protected.

Tides Have Changed

For years, hospitals have been audited for patient care in the facility. If the care was not deemed acceptable or the appropriate level of care because documentation did not support the care, or if the coding was incorrect, then the hospitals would lose the payment for that stay. Medicare would audit and take the money back from the hospitals, not the physicians. You were not financially impacted even though your documentation was very important to the success or failure of the claim. That has now changed. And a critical problem for most physicians is they are not documenting in a way that protects them later from being audited.

Data Mining

Medicare has started data mining all of your bills against

the outcomes of your patients to determine what kind of reimbursement you will get. They are positioning for a change in 2015 when they will start auditing your charts and begin taking money back from both hospitals and physicians. They have made a new rule that allows them to go back as far as five years. In other words, if they find a pattern of discrepancy, starting in 2015 they can audit you as far back as 2010, and take money back.

I know I sound like a broken record in repeating how and when they can take your money back, but this is the new reality. You need to be fully aware of this and begin documenting properly NOW.

Know that Medicare is currently data mining everyone, and in 2014 will put into effect who they will audit first in 2015.

Remember, they are the government, and with the upcoming enrollment surge of baby boomers, they need to take money back in an effort to prepare for the expenses. If your charts are not complete, or not accurate, or not reflecting the required Medicare language necessary, then you will be a target for audit... and they will take back money already paid to you.

What They Look for When Auditing Your Charts

Medicare auditors are looking to see if you have supporting documentation. They are looking for over-utilization. For example, a few years ago there was a period where physicians were documenting sepsis on almost every patient that came in if they had an elevated heart rate and an elevated temperature. But, you can have an elevated heart rate and an elevated temperature with a cold. That does not necessarily mean the patient has sepsis. Therefore sepsis became a target diagnosis. Medicare started looking at every sepsis bill that was submitted because they found that too many physicians were using that diagnosis.

When you see that you are over-utilizing a diagnosis, then you may not be documenting appropriately. Sepsis is not appropriate for someone with a cold. It is appropriate for someone with an elevated white count, heart rate, respiration rate and temperature. With those symptoms, you can now tell Medicare that the patient is septic. Next, can you say that the patient is in septic shock? Well, that depends. Are they in a life-threatening situation? Do you have to give them four liters of fluid? Have you determined what source the sepsis is coming from? Is it coming from pneumonia? Or what else? It is really important to document the symptoms fully and appropriately.

Every physician I have ever known does everything in his or her power to take care of their patient. The problem is, since Medicare has now changed the rules, you must paint a literal picture of the patient lying in that bed.

Previously, you could simply write something like, "patient unstable, continue current treatment, add this medication and add that lab" and you would be done. Medicare no longer finds this acceptable.

Now you must say, "I have a sixty-five year old female with diabetes, CAD, is in Stage III renal disease and doesn't free on dialysis, came in with elevated WBC, hypertension, low blood pressure, with a heart rate of 130."

Now, with this last instance, I *painted a picture* of a patient who could very well be in the ICU. That's what Medicare is looking for.

HIGH COST OF APPEALS

We are faced with more audits today than ever before and many hospitals are now paying out millions upon millions of dollars in appeals each year. The expenses incurred to fight an audit are colossal. Currently, the average hospital has $3 million to $10 million dollars a month in appeals on their plate from Medicare alone. And with the odds stacking in Medicare's favor, those numbers are projected to go higher.

According to the 2012 HHS Agency Financial Report, an estimated $31.2 billion in improper payments will be paid in 2013. They have stated, "The primary causes of improper payments, as identified in the Medicare FFS Improper Payments reports, are insufficient documentation errors, medically unnecessary services, and to a lesser extent, incorrect coding."

In the medical legal world, if it didn't get written it didn't happen. Improper documentation can result in litigation. It's important to have your documentation written in a codeable language that is acceptable by government standards. This makes your entire litigation easier to fight because it will show the entire picture of the patient, the care provided and that you followed best practice with your care, thus helping you to avoid litigation in the first place.

Five Levels of Appeals

The levels of appeal are posted on the web site of Centers for Medicare and Medicaid Services, http://www.CMS.gov .

1) First Level of Appeal: Redetermination by a Medicare carrier, fiscal intermediary (FI), or Medicare Administrative Contractor (MAC).

2) Second Level of Appeal: Reconsideration by a Qualified Independent Contractor (QIC)

3) Third Level of Appeal: Hearing by an Administrative Law Judge (ALJ) in the Office of Medicare Hearings and Appeals

4) Fourth Level of Appeal: Review by the Medicare Appeals Council

5) Fifth Level of Appeal: Judicial Review in Federal District Court

In other words, for each one of those appeals, you have to employ someone to go back through the records, prepare it, copy it, and then send it off to be reviewed. *Ka-ching!* If it doesn't pass the first level of appeal, it goes to the second level of appeal where you have to hire an outside agency to start writing your appeal for you. *Ka-ching! Ka-ching!* If it doesn't pass the second level, then it goes to the third level; you have to hire an attorney to fight for you. *Ka-ching! Ka-ching! Ka-ching!*

You get the drift.

Clinical Review Judgment

Just this last year, CMS has added a new layer to the appeals process, which created another dimension to the first level of appeal that you have to go through before you can receive your money back. RAC now uses Clinical Review Judgment (CRJ) when they think the medical record does not support the clinical diagnoses. What this means is if they don't find your record as accurate in documentation, they are going to look for clinical indicators to make sure that you have listed your clinical indications for every diagnosis. RAC using CRJ started in Boston, MA and is now rolling out throughout the entire country.

Once you have submitted your medical records, it is reviewed and questions might arise. If they are not sure that you have met all of your clinical indicators, it will now go through a new layer of review, which is clinical validation. It is here that you must spell out each component, such as the difference between SIRS, sepsis, and septic shock. Understanding the difference between what those three levels are and being able to speak to them is exactly what they will be looking for.

If you were to have a patient that comes in with SIRS, they would generally have an elevated white count, heart rate, possibly elevated temperature and low blood pressure. When they go into true sepsis, you would need to determine if an organism such as staph or MRSA exists in order for you to treat them with a broad-spectrum antibiotic. However, if it is septic shock, your patient will probably be in the ICU, have to receive a fluid challenge of more than 4 liters in an hour, and be considered clinically unstable.

Being able to distinguish between these different levels is what clinical validation is all about.

Going forward, it is imperative that you are very specific and ***paint a clear and concise picture of each diagnosis*** using all information that is available for clinical validation.

What About Fines? Penalties? Interest?

As of the date of this book, Medicare has not made a clear determination or announcement whether there will be fines, penalties or interest charged on the monies taken back. In the past, we have seen them fine institutions and take money back due to a perception of fraud. We are currently unaware of the actions they will take. However, I can tell you what I believe. Based both on the way the government works and from my experience, we will be seeing large fines attached.

Reasons for Proper Documentation

There are five reasons proper documentation is more important today than ever before.

1) Physician Profiling

2) Pay for Performance (P4P)

3) Preparation for ICD-10

4) Value-Based Purchasing

5) The RAC and other Audit Claw Backs

Proper documentation is important to protect you in many ways; not only with Medicare looking at your charts, but with any family that is upset and takes you to court. Two years from now, you may or may not remember everything that had happened. But if you can **paint a complete picture** for yourself, you will be able to pick up this chart at a later date, understand the case, and fully explain what happened because of your appropriate documentation. It helps in the transitions of care. It means that your patient gets treated at the appropriate level at the appropriate time, which then makes you a better provider in the eyes of Medicare (as well as everyone else).

This will also make you a better provider to that patient. That patient will then feel that you have cared for them, talked to them, and that you have helped them transition from one level to the next.

The other factor to consider is that, with a lawsuit, you have something specific to look back on. In a Medicare audit you can back your diagnosis with your documentation, allowing you to get that appeal overturned. You have the right to appeal. Proper documentation protects you in today's world as well as in the world to come.

What's Next?

So you've faced the RAC audits, you've faced the appeals, and you feel like winning isn't possible. If all of that has you scared and you are still reading this book, then I commend you. You truly are a fighter. You are ready to position yourself by knowing what is coming and how to train for it. In addition to the changes on how you document, there is also a new electronic world coming, and in order to conquer it, we must bring our A-Game and fight to win.

So let's go!

Mark Kimmel, Ph.D.

Chapter 3

The New Electronic World

In the ever-changing world of medicine, the new electronic world has arrived with Medicare's decision that, by 2015, all medical records must be electronic. This changes the way we practice medicine. Before, you could write three lines, order a test and you'd be done. Now, every time you see a patient, you must ask specific questions related to the care of that patient. It is much more involved. In this chapter we will explore some of those changes and how you can get ahead of this game.

ALL MEDICAL RECORDS
MUST BE ELECTRONIC

Effective January 2015, the Health Information Technology for Economic and Clinical Health (HITECH) Act mandates that medical records must be made electronic. Everyone is going to have to prove outcomes. And you can only prove outcomes in two ways: one is by your patients' results, and the other is with your documentation.

Part of Medicare's problem is that they are getting hundreds of thousands of pieces of paper, including faxes. There is always human error. Papers get lost. Faxes get jammed. And there will be appeals and re-appeals when information is not received.

With a digital PDF file, they are unable to say that they are missing any of the parts. They won't be able to claim that something wasn't sent. This will streamline the process and make it less painful because only one complete set of documents will be sent at one time. In summary, they are moving to electronic filing due to both cost and efficiency.

The Independent Practice Association (IPA) will also need an electronic medical record with the same guidelines or else they too will lose their funding from the federal government. As you can see this affects independent physician groups and well beyond the hospitals and universities because you will have to show effective documentation as well as documenting electronically; this is all a new concept.

This is a complete change in healthcare.

One thing that Medicare has learned in its 48 years of existence is that continuity is key. They know that if there is a nationally accessible electronic medical system, there will soon be a way to link all medical records together, thus giving a complete picture of a patient, no matter where they are.

For people who value privacy, this can be very disconcerting. But as a healthcare provider myself, I can't tell you the number of times patients would come into the ICU unable to give us their history. They couldn't tell us what medications they were taking; it was like shooting in the dark trying to help them. You can do your best to take care of a patient, but you can't offer them optimal care if you are unable to view their history.

Now that we have moved into an electronic world, it is easier to view a chart's PDF file rather than sort through a thousand pages of paper. Medicare will then run programs with your NPI number to identify patterns or tracks and trends. If you have an electronic medical record, it is easier for them to create a program to scan your records and ensure that you are doing the right thing.

It is now more important than ever that we get this right. The reality is that we have moved from cardex to computer, computer to electronic documentation, and now to the point where this is not just a proposed idea, but a requirement. In this ever-changing world, we must be prepared to make these changes, and make them efficiently.

YOUR NPI NUMBER

You have an NPI number. Do you know why? Do you understand how this is linked to how you get paid? Do you know how this will determine your ranking as a physician?

In 1996, the Health Insurance Portability and Accountability Act (HIPAA) was enacted. As part of this, in 2006, every healthcare provider in the United States was issued a National Provider Identifier (NPI) number. There is a national registry for the NPI number, which was made available on September 4, 2007 and can be accessed online.

Once an NPI number is issued, it is permanent regardless of circumstances like a job or location change. Regardless of whether or not a healthcare service bills insurance companies, it is still mandatory that they have an NPI number. This is the way you are identified.

Your NPI number is attached to an electronic format in which Medicare compiles data about you. The world we live in today is completely different. Previously, everything was written on paper and was very short and to the point. But by 2015, every provider in the United States will be required to have an electronic format.

Taxonomy Codes

Attached to the NPI number is a taxonomy code. Taxonomy Codes are administrative codes set for identifying the provider type and area of specialization for healthcare providers. They are alphanumeric and are ten characters in length. Taxonomy codes allow providers to identify their specialty. A provider can have more than one taxonomy code.

Taxonomy Codes have three distinct levels:

Level I: Identifies the provider type, which is a major grouping of healthcare providers. For example: Dentists, Osteopathic Physicians, and Chiropractors.

Level II: The classification or a more specific service or occupation related to the provider type.

Level III: The Area of Specialization. This is a more specialized area of the classification in which a provider chooses to practice or make services available. This is usually based upon the sub-specialty certificate.

Taxonomy Codes allow the provider to identify their specialty at the claim level. This can directly affect your reimbursement from insurance companies. In other words, if you have an inaccurate taxonomy code linked to your NPI number, then your services may be paid at a lower reimbursement rate, or outright denied by an insurance company.

Your Ranking Publically Reported

In 2015, the NPI will become a publically reported number. As a result you will be ranked based on the claims submitted and the accuracy of those claims to determine what type of provider you are. More than likely, it will be similar to the hospital ratings with 1-5 Stars ranking from poor to good. What this means is that you can be the best doctor in the world, but if you don't know how to document in the government's language, you will be ranked as a poor provider.

As you know, the world has become digital and anyone can look you up on the Internet. They will be able to see how you are ranked and with whom you are affiliated. Medicare will be putting this out, and based upon your billing component, you will be ranked from a good to poor provider.

Due to the implementation of the NPI number as part of the HIPAA Compliance Act, a database was compiled of every physician, and every bill, and everything that is associated with these through Medicare. So, if you are a Medicare provider submitting a bill, whether it is through a health plan, a facility, or your office, everything you have done has been saved in a database.

You are then ranked based upon the data that you have

submitted on your bill. This information will then be posted publically on the Internet. So everything about your Medicare practice and your outcomes are going to be publically reported.

For Example

If you have a patient who comes in and dies unexpectedly, that death gets contributed to you as the provider. Now, there are ways to make sure that that death is contributed correctly. If you have a patient who comes in with metastatic cancer and you put them on comfort measures, a morphine drip and then they die, you have to write (and be sure that your coders code) that your patient was on hospice comfort care. In your documentation, you have to specifically say, "This outcome is expected. The patient expired on such-and-such. The patient was on comfort care for such-and-such." If you do not state that this was an expected outcome AND make sure that your bill was coded with that comfort care diagnosis, then that death is contributed to you.

What does that mean? You can give the right care to the right patient at the right time, but if you do not document it appropriately, their death will be counted against you, and that gets publically reported.

Viewing Your Ranking Online

You can check on any provider by going to:
https://npiregistry.cms.hhs.gov.

By entering the provider's name, city, and state you will be able to see license numbers, NPI numbers and Medicare provider numbers. Soon you will see a ranking for each provider that will appear by Medicare based on claims data.

Why is this important? Because this will be the way you are paid by health plans. This is what patients, hospitals, IPA's and any other employers will look for. If your documentation does not support the care you provided to a patient then Medicare, health plans and others will claim potential fraud. You can be the best provider in the world, however, if you do not document in a codeable language, you are then at a great disadvantage.

How to Help Your Ranking

There is currently no state of appeal for the ranking. However, you can appeal the bill. That means if your bill was audited and they find that things were not coded properly, you can have it resubmitted. That is your only route of appeal at this time.

To help ensure that your ranking is accurate, constantly monitor and review your documentation to make sure that you are documenting properly. Then, have a reputable coding service to submit the bill for you. It is very important what appears on that bill. Not only should the numbers be correct, but you must have full documentation that supports the level of care, the severity of illness, the diagnostic tests and medications that you are giving to them.

For Example

If you have a patient that comes in with chest pain and you find out that they have GERD, yet continue on a cardiac path, you won't get paid. If you then change your diagnosis to GERD, do an EGD and start the patient on a PPI, you can get paid. It is very important to understand your patient, understand what you are documenting and understand what Medicare is looking for.

To better impact your ranking now, work with your coders and CDI specialist to improve your documentation.

Currently, if your facility does not use an electronic format, you need to start that process. Because at this point, Medicare has already changed the game and the burden is on you to play catch up. If you don't move now, in 2014 all of your bills will be scrutinized. For every pattern found, you will be audited. When 2015 arrives, they will start taking money back from you. **You must start now.**

Begin studying and start the learning process. Pay attention to the information that is around you. We can send you helpful tips on what is happening in the Medicare arena. We can send you a blast on what their current targets are. We can help you get the information in a format that is easy for you to digest.

TEMPLATE FOR NOTES

When thinking about designing a template for a note, you must keep several things in mind such as CMS guidelines and whichever regulatory agency that you use, such as Joint Commission on the Accreditation of Healthcare Organizations (JCAHO), and their quality measures. This means that your notes may look a bit longer and may seem a bit cumbersome, but with the proper structure, the note can be quick, easy and efficient, and give you a total package within one document.

As previously stated, in this new electronic world, our notes have changed as our medicine has changed. Every time Medicare, CMS, JCAHO or any other regulatory agency makes a change, you must document to those changes. Therefore, this is another evolving document that must be continually updated based on the changes sent out by Medicare, CMS or JCAHO regulations.

The consequences of not complying with this are going to be multi-factorial:

1) There will come a time when you will not be able to see Medicare patients or Medicare Advantage patients if you do not have an EMR. Of course, exceptions will be addressed for those not in Internet accessible areas.

2) Another issue with not having an EMR is that your note is much harder to defend. With a handwritten note, they can simply write back, "Unable to read submitted documentation." Then you could lose that entire stay. With an EMR, they are unable say that they can't read it. You will now have eliminated a reason for denial.

3) The possible outcomes and variances are decreased when you have a standardized note. If you are asking the same questions about every patient, you are more apt to get into a pattern of asking those specific questions that are laid out by Medicare, CMS, JCAHO or any other regulatory agency. It will become second nature for you because you will know how to answer them.

4) Finally, you will be able to utilize components that make the patient special or more difficult to deal with. Then, specificity can be used to your advantage. From answering all of those questions necessary to meet requirements, you then can **_paint the picture_** of how sick this patient is in an electronic format more quickly

than you can in writing.

This is important because every point in an electronic record becomes a data point. Not only is it important for review by Medicare, but in many ways it will benefit you as well. Reports can be created in the back of your system that will allow you to see details of your patients and give you a better understanding of your population. As a physician, it will help you in knowing where to concentrate on education and what the upcoming new treatments are for your patients. In addition, it will allow you to become more adaptable to the changes in your particular population.

We tend to treat patients antidotically and have an understanding of the number of patients we have, but there might be patients that do not come to the forefront of your mind. However, when you can write a report on a specific diagnosis or treatment that seems to be reoccurring, you then can look for answers to help in treatment of that diagnosis and find all patients that fall within that diagnosis.

Remember, in this new electronic age, data is going to become one of your points of defense. Why data? Because you can statistically prove the high-risk nature of your patients and the need for the care you validate as well as the need for money spent on treatment. You will also be able to prove the outcome with improved quality of life and the appropriate transition of care.

Data will always show you areas of weakness in your systems. Data will help you target upcoming trends in healthcare. Review of denials will help you stay in front of the coming wave of change.

Your data will become one of your best friends.

HOW TO IMPLEMENT

When you implement your note, you need someone who understands your electronic system as well as Medicare, CMS and JCAHO guidelines. This can help you answer a series of questions specifically designed to meet those guidelines. It gives you a defensible note. It also gives you clear and concise data points.

When you begin implementing your EMR, there are several important points such as remembering the rules and regulations provided by CMS. In building your note ensure that you answer key questions such as why the patient needs to be an inpatient versus an outpatient. Once you have established those questions and implemented them in your note, you will have the ability to pull clear, clean and concise data.

One of the many current quality measures for patients being admitted into a hospital is Deep vein thrombosis (DVT) or Venous Thromboembolism (VTE). Medicare is now looking at these measures. If your patient is not put on VTE prophylaxis and they develop a DVT while in the hospital, you will not be paid for the care of that patient.

These statistics also become a part of your ranking that is attached to your NPI number. All of these components are intermingled. And in order to implement this, you have to look at what measures and standards you are being held accountable. Then, you have to put this into Medicare's acceptable coded language. Your best defense is to communicate in codeable language. You may have your own way of saying it, but if you don't meet Medicare guidelines, you are not documenting appropriately and this will lead to trouble for you down the road.

A NOTE OF CAUTION:
DO NOT USE *copy forward* or *copy and paste.*

This has become a hot button issue that can result in an audit. Even if your plan does not change a lot from day to day, Medicare is very clear that you must document a complete new note on a daily basis. Many systems will allow you to pull in labs or vital signs for a few days to trend (and that is good), however on a daily basis, DO NOT allow your plan from the note to pull in from the prior note.

KNOW WHO'S WATCHING YOU

Several agencies are in place for three primary reasons: to protect the patient, reduce fraud and take back money if you do not support the need for care. All of these organizations are looking at your outcomes and ultimately report to the Office of Inspector General (OIG). This is a cabinet level position that reports directly to the President of the United States regarding its issues. What this means to you is that your simple Medicare bill has a link directly up to Congress and to the President.

At that level, everything is scrutinized. As a provider, you want to ensure that you are giving the appropriate care, at the appropriate level, for the appropriate length of time to ensure optimal outcomes. This is just like a lean process in any business. Basically, Medicare has taken parts of lean and has applied it to medicine. Any process that can be repeated can be made into a lean process. As you know, in process, that is good, but in patient care it doesn't necessarily work.

With patients, there are so many variables that it is almost impossible to create a true lean process. We've created standards of care, which say that a patient with a specific diagnosis should be treated for a certain number of days. However, that doesn't always apply to every patient because they have different risks factors.

I am sure that you have heard a lot of chatter in the medical community about the recovery audit contractors, known as RAC. Their sole purpose is to review your charts and bills to ensure that you have given the correct care, at the correct time, at the correct level, and for the correct duration. On the downside, they get paid a percentage. In other words, they receive a percentage of every Medicare dollar that they get refunded from you. So they are highly-motivated to get money back from you.

From my perspective, that seems a little unfair. But again, we didn't make the rules; we just have to play by them.

The need to document appropriately is becoming one of the primary focuses for every healthcare provider in the United States. Knowing what is "expectable" or what is in "codeable language" will impact every aspect of your work. With your every move being reviewed by so many agencies, the need to support your work is now a requirement for success.

Here are the top agencies and audits you need to be aware of:

Comprehensive Error Rate Testing (CERT)

Department of Justice (DOJ)

Health Care Fraud Prevention and Enforcement Action Team (HEAT)

Improper Payments Information Act (IPIA)

Medicaid Integrity Contractors (MICs)

Medicaid Integrity Program (MIP)

Medicare Administrative Contractor (MMA)

Office of Inspector General (OIG)

Payment Error Rate Measurement (PERM)

Program Safeguard Contractors (PSC)

Recovery Audit Contractor (RAC)

Zone Program Integrity Contractors (ZPIC)

(NOTE: You'll find short descriptions of these agencies in the index at the back of this book. If you would like further information, all of these agencies can be found online.)

CONSEQUENCE OF NON-COMPLIANCE

I can't say it enough that the consequences of non-compliance are multi-factorial. There are solid reasons why:

1) You won't have the data to support your outcomes.

2) You won't have a way to track and trend what is happening with your particular practice.

3) You won't know how many patients you are treating for any particular diagnosis.

4) All of the information issued to Medicare through your NPI number comes from what you have documented and submitted on your bill.

5) You won't know your gaps in care or systems without data.

If you don't comply with the requirement of electronic medical records, the consequences can change the course of your career. You will receive a lower ranking with Medicare; you will most likely lose your appeals if you are audited, and by 2015, you will be fined for every year you do not have electronic medical records. Eventually, if you are not in full compliance, you will no longer be permitted to treat patients that are Medicare or Medicare Advantage.

The consequences of your actions are tantamount to your success. It's your choice whether you step up and do what is necessary. Keep in mind the consequence of non-compliance is failure, thus not allowing you to provide for your family and greatly affecting your lifestyle if you do not succeed.

The consequences are THAT BIG.
You must take them seriously.

POSSIBLE OUTCOMES AND VARIANTS

One thing that your electronic medical record does is to help you prove your outcomes. How is that? Each patient is ranked on the health scale based upon his or her morbidity rate. Your documentations are the only way Medicare can assess the morbidity rate that factors in how much money you are paid for the care you give. Their outcomes depend heavily upon your documentation. Your variant components will answer what is wrong with that patient.

What if you were to have forty patients that have two or

three diagnoses and you have ten patients that have twenty diagnoses? With this, you have a big variance. How do you know their sickness levels by what you are documenting?

Remember, Medicare cannot see your patients; they can only see your documentation.

NEED TO STATISTICALLY SUPPORT YOUR WORK

All of your variances and outcomes are statistical points. You need to *paint a picture* for Medicare in your documentation and statistically support what is happening.

If you have forty patients with one diagnosis, twenty patients with another diagnosis and 20% of your patients are very high risk needing the most care, you must determine what you can do to help them. These outcomes support your work.

For Example

Mrs. Brown is admitted to the hospital because she is short of breath from fluid overload. She can't get up and walk due to peripheral vascular disease and she can't feel her feet. You know it's going to take longer for her to get better because one of the interventions for congestive heart failure is ambulation along with Lasix, to help remove the fluid. But if she is unable to walk, that's going to slow down her progression. It's going to take longer for her to get better. But Medicare is unable to see that if you only tell them you are treating the CHF. If you don't tell them about the other factors that are keeping that patient in the hospital, or keeping that patient from progressing in best practice, they will hold you responsible and rank you as a bad physician.

In other words, this can all be used to statistically support your work. In order to do that, you must have a way to gather the information. Your EMR then becomes not only a way for you to get paid, but it also supports the work that you are doing. Every standard statement within your medical record can become a statistical point.

At the end of the month you can run a report on your patients to determine how many are critically ill, how many are stable and how many are healthy. You can then work with your health plan to negotiate. For example, if the health plan is only paying you for ten high-risk patients, but you can prove that you have twenty-nine, you will be able to support this with numbers to back it up.

Corporations work specifically on statistics. If you statistically support what you want to accomplish, then you can make changes.

When I worked in a large health organization, we wanted to add a new clinic. In order to do so, we had to prove the need for that clinic. The only way we could prove the need was to pull information and present numbers. We needed to show numbers on patients that had been readmitted, the costs for those readmissions and our costs to send those patients out and have them come back in again. We had to present these numbers to *paint a picture* for the administration of the facility. Once that was done, they understood the organizational impact and were more willing to add the clinic. Although a clinic had been discussed for five years, they were unwilling to spend the money until we could present them with supported information that they could understand.

The same thing applies for Medicare. If you can

statistically support the level of care needed to take care of your patients, you can then get paid for that level of care. This is why it is necessary to have supporting documentation and data.

Medicare states it would appear that you are committing fraud if you don't support what you are doing. You can move yourself away from the fraud category by statistically supporting what you are doing and documenting appropriately.

What Medicare Defines as Fraud

Medicare's definition of fraud now includes any deviance from standard practice or anything you bill that is not documented.

For Example

A patient comes in with acute chest pain; you diagnose them with COPD, and treat them for COPD. However, if you haven't documented what was done and that bill gets sent in with COPD, you have potentially committed fraud. Understand that it isn't because you didn't treat your patient; it is due to the fact that you didn't document the cause. If your charts get audited and you haven't documented properly, although you might be the best physician to have ever existed, you would appear as a substandard provider.

Look at the simple fact that, as a provider, you will review a checklist in your mind when you see this 78-year-old patient with diabetes, hypertension, cardiovascular disease and peripheral vascular disease. However, looking at this picture, if you only document, "Patient came in with chest pain, low potassium." you haven't *painted that picture* for the reviewer. In other words, when they review the chart and see that you have given the patient Lasix, you've performed a Doppler, started them on Coreg, but didn't document **WHY** you did these things, Medicare will consider this to be possible fraud.

It isn't that you are not a good physician; it isn't that you are not providing the right care; it's just that you are not documenting appropriately. Again, if the bill is submitted without the supporting documentation, Medicare views that as potential fraud.

There are measures you can take to ensure that you are not committing Medicare fraud. A good way is to get a reputable coding company or organization that can help you. Although, there are a lot of people who say that they can code for you, what is their background? What is their rating? How do they know what they know? Working with an automated system can help you, and then having the balance of a complete CDI team can save you millions. Of course, that is going to cost money to get set up, however what it can save you in the long run is enormous. When you consider that the average physician gets paid $100 thousand to $300 thousand dollars a year from Medicare for seeing patients in their office, and can be paid up to $1 million dollars for seeing patients in the hospital, all of this is now going to be at risk going back as far as five years starting in 2015. The small investment you make now could save you millions.

Keeping Up With the Changes

The problem is that Medicare is so large and it may look like there is no way to win. This is understandable since we are in a game that is fixed in their favor. But there is a solution! Together we can win! And anything worth winning is worth fighting for.

As you know, spending time with your patients is very important. Although every provider doing his or her documentation in an electronic format that may ultimately be saving time, the path to get there is not. The transition needs to be made. You must be able to understand what is needed in the note, get it done as quickly as possible, use as much of a point-and-click that answers your question, and then have it written in a format and a language that is accepted by Medicare.

There is a lot of information about Medicare fraud and the electronic age, but the point I am really stressing is that we are in an ever-changing world that may seem difficult to keep up with. It may seem insurmountable for you as a provider to keep up with these changes, still care for your patients, and work to balance all this with your personal life.

These changes affect all of us mentally and emotionally. Yet, if you've made it this far, and as you position yourself into a manageable situation with a tool like Codeable Language™, you will be able to thrive in the new digital age.

Chapter 4

Trends and Predictions

Keeping up with the changes as well as the trends in our industry and using the available tools puts you on the forefront of your own success. Your best friend is data, data, and more data. This may seem insurmountable, but it is important to your success.

Reading periodicals and connecting with a large network of colleagues and friends are some of your best ways to gather information. Medicare sends out weekly blasts giving you updates. Periodicals, such as "Society of Hospital Medicine" send information about the turnings of tides and the current changes. The RAC updates will present information about what is occurring. There is plenty of information out there for you to obtain.

Another way to stay current, specific to you and your practice, is to review your charts. Do a review of your audits. Sit down with the hospital administration and go over all of the charts denied. Look at Medicare's reasons for denying. Having someone on your team who can interpret this information and give you accurate feedback is invaluable for winning at this point in the game.

If you have thirty charts and seven of them are being audited for one particular diagnosis, you can be sure that someone else around the country is being audited for the same thing. Tapping into that network throughout the United States to see what it is being targeted allows you to build your defense before you get audited on those particular items.

Riding the Wave of Change

You'll want to make available to yourself the ability to track the trends and stay ahead of what's happening. Just as in surfing, you analyze a wave as it swells and paddle perfectly into position as it begins to break. This is where you want to be. You don't want to be at the bottom of the wave and have it crash down on you. You want to see from the beginning as Medicare starts changing their targets and protect yourself by ensuring your documentation is in full compliance.

Take a good look at all of the claims data and analyze it. Look at all of the available information to follow trends. Monitor your documentation to make certain that it will fully withstand an audit. Foresight allows you to be prepared and gives you the advantage to see when Medicare is changing the target diagnosis. Then, along with proper documentation, you will paddle into position and ride your wave to success.

RAC CHANGING OF THE TARGET DIAGNOSIS

When RAC sees a large amount of bills coming through on a particular diagnosis, they choose that diagnosis as a target.

They will then start auditing those bills to see if there is a trend occurring throughout the United States. They are looking to see if providers document appropriately and admit at the proper level of care. They will use data mining through your NPI number and the claims you submit to find possible target areas.

While tracking what the RAC is saying, we noticed the trends for abdominal pain. So we went through all of the charts that they were pulling for the pre-audits and noticed that pneumonia and abdominal pain were their targets. We started looking at our documentation. We identified what was occurring with these particular items. We were then able to build a strong claim and were much more prepared to defend these audits.

Today, supporting documentation, clinical indication and medical need for the level of care is in Medicare's scope of targets. There is a lot of emphasis on whether a patient should be treated inpatient or outpatient. In this area alone, they have moved some seventy-six diagnoses from inpatient to outpatient.

Now that people are anticipating the criteria that Medicare will be auditing, Medicare is changing their targets every four to six months. Being able to forecast the next trends is truly an art. Plain and simple, it's an educated guess based on information compilation and fact.

TRACKING AND TRENDING DATA

Medicare is constantly changing the target diagnosis. If you understand this, you can then structure your note to speak to their questions. When you receive a pre-audit request for charts, look at what they are specifically asking. Look at how many charts and diagnoses are being pulled. This can help you to track and trend the upcoming diagnosis. You can accomplish this by simply dissecting this information and doing a statistical analysis.

For Example

If you have forty charts that are pulled, ten are on a single diagnosis, ten are on mixed diagnoses, and twenty are on a particular diagnosis like abdominal pain, then you can see that abdominal pain is their current target.

If the trend is abdominal pain, you then want to make certain that your closing diagnosis is not abdominal pain. But remember, abdominal pain is a target diagnosis. Appendicitis, GI bleed and GERD all fall under abdominal pain. So, your final diagnosis should be the cause of that abdominal pain. For years, we used a symptom like abdominal pain as a diagnosis, however, it is not codeable language and can no longer be billed as such (exception: there is no underlying cause for the abdominal pain). You can have unspecified abdominal pain, but the payment on it is very low. The more you specify and properly document, the better you will be paid. Your documentation now must speak to Medicare's required language.

Medicare Looking for Level of Care to Match Diagnosis

Along with data mining for diagnosis trends, Medicare is also looking for the level of care to match the diagnosis.

If you have a patient who comes in with shortness of

breath and no other symptoms, that should be an observation, unless the patient has an underlying symptom that requires inpatient care. Understand that in documenting your need for the level of care, you must list the risk to that patient if they go home. List what can't be done in an outpatient setting, what can be done in an inpatient setting, and what your fears are if this patient were to go home. *Paint the full picture.*

Medicare is looking to see if you have documented enough to support inpatient, or if you only documented enough to support outpatient. If you don't give enough supporting documentation for inpatient, you will be down coded to ambulatory services, which is a lower payment.

UNDERSTANDING THE OUTCOMES

Every time you receive a denial from Medicare, it is important to understand why you were denied and whether you have sufficient documentation to appeal.

A simple denial to understand would say, "Unable to Read Physician Documentation." If they are unable to read your note, you have no basis to appeal. The rules and regulations state that the documentation must be clear. If the physician's handwriting is not legible to the masses, they can deny your claim. This is why it is important to have an electronic medical record.

However, if you get a denial that states it is the wrong level of care, then you need to know what to search for in this chart. Is there supporting documentation that states why this should have been treated as an inpatient? Or not? Is there sufficient documentation that supports your fears in sending the patient home? Or not? For each type of appeal, you need to look for specifics in the patient's chart.

NAVIGATING APPEALS

Okay... now you have received your RAC results and ten charts were denied... your heart sinks and you let out a sigh of defeat. You know that you did the work; you documented to the best of your knowledge, yet you are not getting paid. It is now your job to go through those charts and find out why you lost those cases.

You may be thinking this is overwhelming and wondering how this can be accomplished...

This is where it is important for you to build your team. You can have some type of clinical personnel, such as a nurse or PA, to evaluate your charts to see if there was a good diagnosis and supporting clinical information. Then start tearing that chart apart and do a root cause analysis. If you feel like you **painted that picture** and you were wrongly found on this particular chart, then it is time to start the appeals process.

As you know, there are multiple levels of appeal. At the first level of appeal with RAC, you must write a letter of response stating that you feel this denial is inappropriate. List all of your concerns and your reasons for these concerns. I highly suggest the letter be written as if it were being submitted at the ALJ level.

Your letter will now be reviewed for redetermination by a Medicare carrier, fiscal intermediary (FI), or Medicare Administrative Contractor (MAC). If you win at this level of appeal, life is good! If not, you will need to take it to the second level for reconsideration by a Qualified Independent Contractor (QIC). Hopefully you will win at this level. If not, you will have to move to the next level.

By the third level, most companies hire an outside firm to file their appeals. A lot of these firms include physicians who have slowed down or retired and work in conjunction with a law firm to fight for you in front of the ALJ.

The ALJ is the legal component where physicians are questioned about their charts. This is the level where most people can win because you are speaking to another physician; you are actually pleading (generally on the phone) about your particular case.

Speaking physician-to-physician is less complicated when you need them to understand specifics. It's easier to explain while speaking to another person than it is to explain on paper. However, still remember they were not there. And no matter how well you explain, memories fade and details get lost. Your chances of winning at this level certainly increases with better documentation on hand.

Be Prepared

Understanding the appeals process, how it works, and what they are looking for is important to the success of your appeal. Remember, if in the RAC audit you are told that they cannot read the physician's documentation, it is a subjective decision with almost no defense. You can leverage your ability to defend your charts by integrating proper documentation in the beginning. As long as your documentation supports the risk and need for your patient, even if the auditors claim wrong level of care, you have a good chance of winning.

It is important to know when it is worth the fight and when it is best to let go. In this digital age and climate of never-ending change, it's worth the fight when you are ready for it on the front end. Knowing the information that Medicare gets through data mining will empower you to stay far ahead of the trends. Start preparing by building your team. It is vital to have an expert in the arena of gathering data to predict patterns with the same data that Medicare uses to predict patterns. With a clinically designed structured note and the implementation of Codeable Language™, you will have the ability to **paint a clear and concise picture** so that if an appeal is necessary, you have a better chance to win at the first level.

PREDICTIONS

As I stated earlier, Medicare is going through a business redesign in order to stay viable. To do that, they must look at ways to cut the costs. As in any smart business planning, they are looking at the road ahead. So should you. And there are things coming down the pike you need to be aware of.

Next Three to Five Years

Very soon, Medicare will stop paying for "futile" care. Palliative and hospice will be paid, but not curative for those who refuse to accept that they are dying. Mark my words, this is coming in the next three to five years. The reason I say this is because Medicare is continuously putting out articles on how 80% of every dollar is being spent on patients in the last eighteen months of life because the patients were not willing to accept that their death was imminent. Medicare cannot sustain this practice with the upcoming surge of Baby Boomers that will be saturating the system. If it is taking 80 cents of every dollar to treat a patient today, can you imagine what the demand will be in the next three to five years? Currently, we have five patients for every one person paying into Medicare. That will soon grow to ten or fifteen for every one person paying in. How can we sustain this at that rate? We cannot.

Most people are uncomfortable when it comes to talking about the circle of life, how life ends, what needs to be done to get ready for death, or even how to accept the diagnosis. In over twenty years of nursing, I have seen that death is the most difficult time for a family because they don't understand it. For patients who are bed-bound, have no quality of life, are simply lying there in pain, many would believe that keeping them alive is the best thing. Is it? The spiritual answer to that is quite personal. But what is the answer monetarily? How can Medicare support this with the number of new patients entering the system?

Navigating the Death Discussion

In my own case, my father was diagnosed with terminal cancer. The physicians tried to convince me of allowing major surgery on him, of which I refused. He would have spent the last six to eight months in pain. My family was different in the respect that years prior to his passing, my father had told us what he did and didn't want. He also had me as a son, who would never allow something that he didn't want. I prepared my family in the best way that I could to understand what was coming. As a family, we discussed what was going to happen. We discussed what the symptoms would be and how we would treat them. We openly talked about it. Because my father was a minister and we had a spiritual belief, death for us was not a sad occasion. Of course, we were all very sad to be losing him physically, yet we were happy to know that when he did die, he would no longer be in pain and we felt he was going to a better place.

In my father's case, as with many others, death is sometimes the greatest healing that can be received, because while those we love may remain with us in body, they are suffering. This is not to say it is okay to just let someone that is viable die, but to truly understand when keeping someone alive at all cost is not the right thing to do.

We all will struggle with this at some time or another. However, with time and education, we can see the validity in allowing those we love to go in peace. This transition from curative care to palliative or hospice may be difficult depending on your spiritual or cultural beliefs. With this being said, as a provider, you will need to begin this conversation much earlier than ever before. As a nation, we are not good at talking about the circle of life, however with the tide of change that is coming, you will need to progress your practice to include this conversation with every adult patient you see. This conversation is much easier to have when you are not standing at the end of your loved one's bed. In my family's case, my father had been very clear. Most families do not want to speak about death and dying. However, we can aid in this by beginning this discussion when a patient is well.

In another personal instance, a drunk driver killed my Godson's biological parents. He was only sixteen months old at the time this took place, and his parents did not have a will. For the family, it took a large amount of money and a great amount of time to get custody of him because his parents were not prepared for death. They seemed pretty young, so death was neither discussed, nor prepared. Being able to navigate the system as a care provider is difficult. Being able to navigate the system as a novice is almost impossible. The difference between these two cases is not just age, but understanding the need for this discussion. I use this example to remind you that death can arrive at any age. Whether it is a young couple building a life or a man who has lived his life, death can arrive unexpectedly at any time. So again I repeat, the best defense is a good offense. Be prepared and discuss your wishes early rather than later.

So, in the next three to five years, count on Medicare to start denying payment on anything that is considered futile or non-curative care. You need to be prepared.

On a smaller scale, we are currently starting to see this occur within the system. I believe that in the next three to five years this will become a large focus because of the number of Baby Boomers that are going to be hitting the system. Does this mean that everyone who has a chronic disease will lose funding for his or her care? No. What it does mean is that Medicare is going to review much closer the possibility of recovery and what the perceived quality of life can be for a patient.

For Example

You have a patient who is End Stage COPD (chronic obstructive pulmonary disease), and being repeatedly admitted to the hospital. You are able to manage the symptoms, but they continue to get worse. As a provider, you have begun the process of discussing hospice or palliative care, and the patient refuses. Medicare can technically deny payment based on the level of care, stating that symptom management could have been offered at a lower level of care. Due to the fact that the patient is receiving symptom management and not curative care, they would win.

In Europe and other parts of the world it is not uncommon that when a patient reaches this point, they are placed on hospice and allowed to die in peace. If they wish to continue care, they either pay for it privately or through a secondary insurance plan, which can get very costly. Most people are unable to afford this.

Here in the United States, we have not moved to this process. I believe that Medicare will adopt this process to stay viable in the system we have today. This will be a large cultural change in the country as a whole. Medicare will be driving this change based on a business model and the understanding to be able to provide care for the large number of people. They have to change the way they are now doing business.

Next Eighteen Months

In the next eighteen months, you are going to see Medicare really dial in to the importance of supportive information. What does this mean to you? Well, here's your documentation. You think you've done a good job. You've explained the patient's condition. But, do you have the supporting documentation? Have you added that EKG into the note? Have you acknowledged the fact that you've ordered the labs for the next day? Have you acknowledged that you've continued to change the medications? Have you acknowledged that the patient has the current lab values and were they actually listed?

Your supporting documentation and validation for the care needed is going to be extremely important in the next eighteen months. Again, when it goes back to inpatient vs. outpatient, they will be looking for clinical documentation to completely support this. Up until this point, it has not been a focus, but there have been many questions asked about it.

After reading many appeals, I believe that they are heading towards a stronger clinical documentation component (e.g. adding lab values, adding medications, adding comorbidities (CC), adding major comorbidities (MCC), determining the patient's risk, etc.). All of these clinical factors are going to be key in these next eighteen months. More and more facilities are going to see denials based upon lack of supporting documentation.

What to Do Now

My recommendation for you now is to start tracking and trending your denial types. Start documenting to a deeper level. Don't have the time? Well, you have to make the time in order to stay viable in the system as it is today and to survive through the upcoming next three to five years. You are going to have to take the time to build a support team. You are going to have to implement tools that can assist you, such as Codeable Language™. You need to be able to take your electronic medical record and put it in a language that is consistent across the board from your primary to your consults, nursing staff, Medicare and other healthcare plans.

It is not a matter of WHEN, because when is NOW. Although on the surface it may look like you have until 2015 or so before you need to implement, the reality is that you don't. With Medicare, there is a rolling sixteen-month period for review. You can be certain that they will take a sixteen month time period before they implement their rules in order to gain a window to view the way you are doing things. That will be the basis by which they will determine how much you will get paid. This is what they are doing now.

Documenting in Codeable Language™ is important because you are going to need consistency across the continuum to be able to support the care. Medicare is already looking at outpatient care. Can you support what you did as an outpatient? Did you order all of the appropriate tests? Did you perform all of the appropriate treatments to prevent that patient from going to the hospital? As a Medicare provider, if you can say "no" to any of these, you will stand a large chance of losing that payment from Medicare.

Medicare is looking for a consistent transition plan, from the first time, as a primary care physician, that you see a patient to the first time that you will see that patient at the hospital in an acute crisis. Am I saying that every time a patient is admitted to the hospital payment will be denied? No. If you haven't proven that 1) you've educated your patient on diet, 2) focused education to their disease process, 3) spoken and written education of all the preventive measures needed to stay out of the hospital... then you are running the risk of losing payment.

Hospitals and healthcare providers across America are looking at the Medicare changes. Every one of them is a target for audit. My common thread throughout this entire book has and will be that proper documentation makes it easier for your success. Documentation is the ONLY defense you have against these audits.

Now is the time to start building your team of people who

can help you such as your CDI (Clinical Documentation Improvement) Specialist and your trained CLS (Codeable Language Specialist) that can help you document in the appropriate language.

You Must Start Now

If you have not started implementation of your electronic medical records, then you are behind the curve. You need to start this immediately. Design a template for your EMR that meets all of the regulations, and start your Codeable Language™ crosswalk with your documentation. Get the help you need.

These steps need to be your primary focus to get prepared and position yourself to win, and continue to win, because you know Medicare will continue to change the game.

Chapter 5

What "They" Are Saying

It is really important that you understand the magnitude of the change that is coming. You have already proven yourself as a fighter by making it this far. Now it is time to start training like a pro. Michael Phelps, the American swimmer, didn't win 22 Olympic gold medals without putting in some work. And he certainly didn't do it alone. He had a trainer, a coach and a team to back him up. He developed a plan, did the work, and in the end, he got the reward. This can happen for you as well.

For the development of Codeable Language™, I had to spend a lot of time doing chart reviews, reading articles, reading updates from Medicare, and digging into the Affordable Care Act itself. Yes, I will say it. I am a nerd. I read every single page. I felt it was vitally important to know what was coming our way. I knew that, as healthcare providers, we were often reactive rather than proactive with the changes and it was becoming near impossible to keep up. Yet, I was determined to get ahead of the game.

To get there, I went through hundreds of articles... blasts

from The Society of Medicine, The American Academy Association of Case Management, JCAHO, JAMA, essentially blast from everybody. I was able to pull all of this information together and do strategic planning by filtering much of the information and simplifying it down into a fairly easy concept.

Throughout this book I have summarized for you what they are saying. And from all of these associations over the last three to five years, the focus has been on RAC and their denials.

TOP CONTRIBUTING EDITORIALS

It is really important for you to stay apprised of all the new changes. Yes, this does require a lot of time and effort. However, in this electronic age, there are ways to make it simpler.

I receive daily and weekly email updates from several periodicals such as "JAMA", "ACMA", "Medicare New England Journal of Medicine", "Today's Hospitalist", "Society of Hospital Medicine" (SHM), and others. They all send me updates on what is current, not just medically, but also the policies that are changing on the whole Medicare revision. Each of these editorials helps me to understand where we are heading and what we have to do.

It is really important for you to stay up-to-date with each one of these. Topline Healthcare will be sending out blasts informing you of the latest updates from Medicare. "SHM" sends the latest changes that have been filed against Medicare for observation stay vs. inpatient stay; different legislation that has been put into place to try and combat some of the issues that we face. Each and every one of these is important to the success of you and your practice.

SUPPORTING ARTICLES

Going forward, I have listed just a few of the articles that support what we have been covering. With each of them, I have given you a brief summary to help educate and stimulate your thought process. Keep an open mind; see the interconnection and how this impacts your career.

(NOTE: In the digital version of this book, available at Amazon.com, the following articles are linked directly to their sources.)

Greater Use of Clinical Validation Puts DRGs at Risk, Turns Queries Upside Down

http://aishealth.com/marketplace/report-medicare-compliance

The arrival of several things that I had predicted is actually validated in this particular article. "AIS Health" discusses how Medicare is now extremely concerned about validation of where, what, when and why. Why is the patient going to be treated as an inpatient vs. outpatient? Why does the patient have to stay inpatient? What is the risk to this patient if they are not treated as an inpatient? Why now, why not outpatient? What is the outcome of your treatment?

This brings me to sequencing. What is sequencing? It is stating that the event began here... then you did this... then this occurred... and finally you did this.

It becomes really important with this documentation component, as you will see further that Medicare is looking at what is done. Whether it is outpatient or inpatient, they are looking to see if the proper care was delivered and whether all of the applicable components were applied to this patient. **Clinical validation of documentation is becoming extremely important!**

Improving Access to Medicare Coverage Act

http://www.acmaweb.org/section.asp?sID=88&mn=mn5&sn=sn5&wpg=ll

In one of the "American Case Management Association" (ACMA) articles there is a discussion about improving access to Medicare Coverage Act. An unintended consequence of moving a Medicare patient to an observation is that they don't meet a three-midnight stay to be able to qualify for skilled care. Although, I personally believe that this rule is antiquated, it is still in effect.

If a patient is placed on observation, then they are converted to inpatient, the time that they spent on observation is not counted in their inpatient days. If you keep them on observation for 48 hours, then admit them for 24 hours, although they've technically met three midnights in the hospital, requirements have not been met under Medicare's inpatient standard.

That means observation care is completely billed as outpatient services. What is truly inpatient only comes out to one day. That patient, technically in the hospital for three days, cannot go to a skilled nursing facility since they were admitted for only one day.

There is new legislation pending before Congress to change this. There are many people who are asking for this rule to be changed. I believe, as we move into the Medicare exchanges, this rule would be waived, as it is currently for most Medicare Advantage plans. But, as it stands for your straight Medicare patients, this rule has a negative outcome and a negative, unintended consequence.

A really important fact to remember is that any patient on observation status does not have the same right of appeal as an inpatient status because they are technically on an outpatient status while receiving care at an inpatient facility.

Access Hospitals Close Due to Audits

http://www.acmaweb.org/section.asp?sID=88&mn=mn5&sn=sn5&wpg=ll

In another article by "AMCA" they reported that two congressmen, one from Missouri and one from California, have submitted a request to amend the 2003 Medicare Act, which created the RAC Audit Contractors. The congressmen believe that the way the law is written, with the RAC contractors getting a percentage of charges held, makes it an unfair process.

There was a senator in Oklahoma who actually filed suit against Medicare because of the closure of three access hospitals in Oklahoma. When our own lawmakers are standing up and fighting because of these changes, we begin to understand the depth in which these changes are occurring.

As an unintended consequence, many hospitals are penalized and have to appeal regardless of whether they are right or wrong. They have no choice but to fight to get their money back. This makes it almost impossible for small access hospitals to be able to survive. Considering that most hospitals work on a 2% margin, if RAC takes back a million dollars, this can close a small hospital. It can reduce the amount of personnel that a medium sized hospital can employ in attempts to offer better care to their patients. If you are a small, independent practitioner, this can completely close your practice and take you out of the game.

CMS Proposed Rule Includes New Medicare Enrollment Restrictions and Measures to Reduce Fraud

http://www.acmaweb.org/section.asp?sID=88&mn=mn5&sn=sn5&wpg=ll

As previously stated in this book, Medicare has redefined fraud to include not being able to clinically support medical care as well as knowingly deceiving the United States government and Medicare. Stated in this "ACMA" article, there is a new proposed rule before CMS currently to increase the penalties and to increase the payout to those who help identify Medicare fraud.

I always say your best defense is a good offense. Your best recourse is to document your patient information appropriately and give that information accurately, in a clear, concise manner. Codeable Language™ will keep you ahead of that. It will allow you a way to document that is clear and exact for your patient and then helps you support the need for their care. You can avoid being put into audit review by documenting appropriately.

How to Steer Clear of the RAC

http://www.todayshospitalist.com/index.php?b=articles_read&cnt=1143&tracking =Site_Search_Results

In this "Today's Hospitalist's" article about how to steer

clear of the RAC, it discusses how to track and trend what is occurring with Medicare. As stated earlier, they recommend that you look at what RAC is currently auditing, such as abdominal pain. And instead of having your final diagnosis be a symptom of abdominal pain, have your final diagnosis come out to be an actual diagnosis such as gastro esophageal *reflux* disease (GERD).

By removing abdominal pain, which is a target for RAC, the chart will not immediately come up for pre-audit bill. They are stating that you need to understand the game, the players in the game and *their* strategy so that you can build *your* strategy to stay ahead.

The Midnight Rule
http://www.regulations.gov/ - !home

There is a proposed change to the Midnight Rule whereas currently a patient on observation will not have their midnights counted until they are placed into the system as an admission.

Brought by CMS there is a new Rule 1599, proposing that the time spent in observation will then count as one of those three midnights and will allow the patient go to skilled care whether they were under observation or were inpatient. This rule will be very beneficial to a lot of senior patients.

It will also remove part of Medicare's payment that is necessary to care for these patients, which is an intended consequence of reducing cost and increasing efficiency. Go to www.regulations.gov and key in Rule 1599.

CMS Allows Rebill

http://www.racsummit.com/resources/Transmittal_1203_Part_B_Inpatient_rebillin g.pdf

Medicare is making some changes in an attempt to reduce the load and impact on hospitals. Currently, if you submitted your inpatient bill and it was denied, you had no recourse if the denial was upheld. However, Medicare has proposed that you can now resubmit that bill under Part B for outpatient services and at least receive some reimbursement for the care that is given to the patient. This is a large change in policy for Medicare and it has very good effects on those who have lost their cases because they now will recoup some money. With the prior implementation, there was no ability for you to recoup any portion of the money. Yes, it is still a net loss, but it is an improvement from where we were before.

Medicare RAC's Take Back $745 Million in Over-payments in the First Quarter of 2013

http://www.beckershospitalreview.com/racs-/-icd-9-/-icd-10/cms-medicare-racs-take-back-745m-in-overpayments-in-1q-of-2013.html

In "Becker's Hospital Review" article we see the financial impact on the industry as a whole due to the RAC audits. In the first quarter of 2013, RAC took back $745 million dollars. That is more than the average income for a large corporation in the United States that Medicare has taken back from the healthcare industry.

Were all of these accurate overpayments? I can't say that is the case. I can say that some of them are, but some of them were due to lack of documentation. If the physicians were able to document the real pictures of the patients, many of these reimbursements would not have been taken back.

Federal EMR Electronic Medical Records Mandate 2014 / 2015 Deadlines http://www.edocscan.com/emr-mandate-2014

As you know, there is a large need for providers to currently have electronic medical records. This "eDocScan" article reinforces that by 2015, if you do not have an EMR, you will start getting a 1% reduction in your Medicare reimbursement. Now, this will be in addition to deductions that are already accrued based upon practice and levels of care. So technically, if you get 1% for not have an EMR and 1% for general reduction for decreased documentation, you could loose 2% of your Medicare reimbursement in the first year across the board. What that means is that on every single Medicare claim you submit, your payment would be reduced by 2% from the beginning. Not cool.

CMS Physician Quality Reporting System
http://www.cms.gov/Medicare/Quality-Initiatives-Patient-Assessment-Instruments/PQRS/Downloads/2013_PQRS_SatisfactoryReporting-Registry_011713.pdf

This CMS article talks about quality measures, and as you know, one of the big pushes from Medicare and CMS is quality outcomes. They're measuring your quality and your DVT's (deep vein thrombosis) that come into your facility, whether they were present on admission or were acquired while they were in the facility.

Under the new payment structure, if a patient has a complication such as a DVT in the hospital that was not present on admission, your payment is reduced and this will go against your quality measures. There are some fifty-eight-quality measures over all, thirteen of which are mandated, three of which are currently being reviewed such as DVT, decubitus ulcer, and urinary sepsis due to catheter placement. These are all being reviewed to determine if they were present upon admission.

Once again, your documentation becomes really important. If a patient comes into your facility with a decubitus ulcer, it is extremely important that you document this. You may ask why? If a patient arrives bedbound, you would expect that they might have some signs of ulcers. But Medicare says that if it wasn't documented by you, it didn't happen. When it is documented by the nurse or the wound care specialist and you failed to document it, they will determine that you did not give appropriate care and that the patient received the decubitus while they were in the facility. This will then lead to you not being paid for the service.

These articles are good on two points: They speak about quality measures and reinforce the fact that Medicare and CMS have built a registry off every single bill that has been submitted. More supporting articles on this subject:

Physician Quality Reporting System:
http://www.cms.gov/Medicare/Quality-Initiatives-Patient-Assessment-Instruments/PQRS/index.html

Quality and Resource Use:
http://www.cardiosource.org/~/media/Files/Advocacy/Physician Payment/2011 QRUR Sample_Cardiology_december 2012.ashx

National Plan and Provider Enumeration System (NPPES)

https://nppes.cms.hhs.gov/NPPES/Welcome.do

This "NPI" article addresses the national registry and its publication. When you read this article you will see that Medicare has clear plans to publish your NPI number along with your contact information, the facility where you work and your ranking. This is the foundation of my talk on how important it is to know what is being submitted in your name and how it is being submitted. This information becomes publically reported in 2015.

MORE GAME CHANGERS

Exchange Program

In the state of California the exchange program has started which is for people who qualify for both Medicare and Medi-Cal (i.e., your Medi-Medi patients). These patients should be your highest paying clientele. However, with the new Affordable Care Act, that will change. HMO patients are going to become more desirable than your Medi-Medi patients because of the way the payment is going to be structured.

Previously with your Medi-Medi patients, you received payment for a portion of the Diagnosis-related Group (DRG), and either Medicaid or Medi-cal (depending on where you live) would pay an additional component of that. With the Medicare restructure, the amount of money being paid on straight Medicare patients is going to be reduced. In essence, Medicare is making it more desirable for patients to move into an HMO system to help control the costs. Therefore, your reimbursement in a Medicare exchange patient will actually be better than that of a straight Medicare patient.

Clinical Validation

Another game changer that has come into play is something I spoke about earlier called Clinical Validation. Speaking with a physician recently, I realized that he was completely unaware of CMS guidelines. As a physician that works for an HMO, he had no idea that clinical validation was necessary on his patients. We were discussing the point of proper documentation and how it needed to be improved. He clearly stated to me, "We get paid a flat rate for our patients, so it doesn't matter what I document." In my mind I thought WHAT? This is not right. So I educated him about clinical validation and documentation using CMS and Medicare guidelines. The look that came over his face was that of total terror. He had been under the assumption that he could simply support his patient HCC scores and have enough validation to get paid.

The game changer is that this may have been true in the past, but that is no longer the case. Your documentation will now directly impact how much you or your organization gets paid for you to care for those patients.

This is a total change in the way that we do business.

If you'll notice, throughout this entire section on supporting data and articles, I have referenced the CMS website and their own blasts being sent out to you as a provider. CMS is trying to get the point across that they are working to calculate every component of what is being done.

When you look at all of these articles, they are talking about the national database and using your NPI number. This is something that I have found most physicians do not fully understand. As a provider, you need to know what is done with your information, how this affects you, how it affects your patients, and ultimately how it affects your ability to provide the best, quality care possible.

Chapter 6

Shifting the Odds in Your Favor

There are many ways for you to shift the odds in your favor. One is by reading book after book, article after article and beginning to formulate your own plan. However, as a provider, this becomes almost an insurmountable task for you to do and still be profitable in what you are doing.

One benefit from reading this book is you will have learned that we have designed and helped implement plans that will put you in front of the game. In a very simple, yet helpful and easy to understand way. I have presented you with information on how to make the most of your electronic medical record, how to properly use your electronic medical record and how to document in Codeable Language™. This way you can run more efficiently and have peace of mind when submitting your note.

We at Topline Healthcare will help you to establish your team. A team is important in business and in play. Your supporting cast at minimum needs to be a CDI Specialist, a Codeable Language Specialist (CLS), a reputable coding company, an expert to help you track and trend all of this data we have discussed, a team that can take all of your appeals and denials and analyze them, do chart review, look at what does and does not work and help you formulate a plan to stay ahead of the game. This is what we do.

To win this game, you must be more strategically placed than ever before.

As you know, the world has completely changed. We have gone from the 1900's to the 2000's in light speed and it may feel like you often can't keep up. We're here to partner with you so that you can meet your optimum goals. We will help you build a viable program. We will make it easy for you to gather and assimilate the data. Then, not only do we fix those areas needing improvement that are identified, but we will also help you do this yourself so you can sustain being ahead of the on-going changes.

As a provider, you have the intellect and the know-how. We respect that the one thing you don't have is the time to dedicate to this and still properly care for your patients. We will come along side, team-up with you and develop a program that will take you from being uncertain to being ahead of the game.

Medicare is not the enemy.

Understandably, you have to fight this battle to win. However, keep in mind that Medicare is trying to accomplish the same goals you are trying to accomplish, just in a completely different way. They are preparing for the wave of baby boomers that will cause a tremendous financial strain on the current healthcare system.

The solution to this is providing a language that calms the beast. One that saves you time and money while helping your patients and giving Medicare what they want. The quickest, most sure way to accomplish these objectives is with the implementation of Codeable Language™.

The solution is education on how to document, what Codeable Language™ is and why it is important to document with it. By implementing our program, your work will not be interrupted by you having to take a six-hour class. Therefore, you won't have to stop what you are doing in your day-to-day practice. This program is an overlay that continually educates you as you are documenting in real-time. It will relieve your stress of wondering if you are doing it right. In one simple step you will understand what Medicare is looking for and what you need to know.

CODEABLE LANGUAGE™ DEFINED

Codeable Language™ is a software tool that has been designed to help you document in the most efficient, complete and accurate way within CMS and Medicare guidelines. It will teach you to document in Medicare approved words and phrases with the appropriate diagnosis and supporting documentation.

The program was designed after many years of experience within the healthcare system and by collecting answers from questions retroactively and repeatedly asked from physicians. This system is designed to ask questions needed at the time of documentation so that you are properly documenting in Medicare's required language and giving them what they want, based on their most current rules and regulations.

In other words, this gives you a document framework needed to meet all of the Medicare guidelines. With all of that in mind, and with the change in healthcare, this system is designed to help you achieve the best outcome possible for your patient.

This helps eliminate problems that arise when communication between providers becomes a gap in the care of a patient. When we are all communicating in the exact same language, this reduces misunderstanding and the need for interpretation.

By using Codeable Language™, you, your colleagues and Medicare are speaking a common language.

As a provider, you have the privilege to help people in some of the most difficult times of their lives. Aside from death, illness is often one of the scariest things that we can face. You are there for people in the beginning of life, during the struggles in the middle, and at the end. You perform a service that no one else can offer. You help bring joy and happiness when delivering a child. You offer comfort during the need for a surgery. And as loved ones are getting ready to pass, you help them transition to Hospice care, giving a dignified and comfortable end to their life. This is a privilege not many people in the world get to experience. Your documentation, in the right language, can help *paint that picture.*

And when you *paint the full picture* of your patients, you and your consultants can provide consistent care, which will lead to better outcomes. Now, when Medicare reviews your chart, they will get a clear, concise and accurate story.

You will be giving them exactly what they are looking for. Everybody is on the same page, speaking the same language, and the common goal to improve healthcare is reached.

How This Program Helps You Document While You Are Working

Codeable Language™ is designed to aid you to document in a language that is acceptable to Medicare, CMS and all current guidelines. The purpose of this is to allow you, as a provider, to document to the highest level without having to spend hours learning and memorizing in a class. As you are documenting with this program, you will receive prompts that will help you learn in real-time. This system was designed with you, the provider, in mind as well as your organization. It was designed to make the transition from paper charts to computerized to a completely codeable documentation in a smooth, effective way without requiring layers and layers of redo. It makes you get it right from the beginning so you don't have to redo it again.

For Example

Let's say that your patient has sepsis. Within the Medicare guidelines, Codeable Language™ tells you what you need to document for sepsis. It will ask you questions that you might not think to address. Is it sepsis due to bacterial pneumonia? Is it sepsis due to CMV pneumonia? The program will then prompt that you need an elevated heart rate, an elevated temperature, WBC's that are above such-and-such, and so on. It tells you signs and symptoms needed to document and support your diagnosis. Therefore, if you are going to document sepsis, this program helps you document all of the points that are necessary to meet Medicare requirements.

This removes you from the labor-intensive abyss of

documentation. It gives you options. And by being specific, you can take a simple diagnosis to a major comorbidity, which will then increase your reimbursement, correctly rank you as a physician, and give the true story of your patient.

WHAT CODEABLE LANGUAGE™ DOES FOR YOU

This program helps you to decrease your costs and time spent while at the same time increase your profitability. It eliminates your need to hire outside help to find out why you are losing so much money through coding. It also eliminates the number of people you need to do the job, which on the bottom line takes away from what you have left to pay in salaries and benefits. It also takes away from what you have left to pay to the government for your match in their social security. So, just from a benefit and wage status alone, you decrease your costs.

For hospitals, you decrease the people you need by automating your system (i.e., instead of having three people review one group of physicians, you could reduce it down to just one who would do retrospective review to ensure accuracy).

Take a look at the three to ten million dollars a month allocated in appeals from Medicare alone. You could potentially reduce this by 80%. How? Because 80% of the denials are based on lack of medical necessity or documentation there of. The Topline Healthcare system, with Codeable Language™, is a complete solution for these issues.

With Codeable Language™ you document and learn in real-time.

You are very busy and don't have the time to sit and take classes, yet you do need to stay updated on the continual changes. No worries, our program helps you learn while you are documenting in real-time.

It will also help you to control and minimize the mistakes. Similar to how Spell Check works to correct spelling errors, Codeable Language™ helps you to increase your documentation skills and improve your status with Medicare by continually reminding you and offering helpful hints in real-time while you are documenting.

How does this help your patients?

Codeable Language™ works on several key components. It helps you as the provider to document everything you have done for your patient and to make sure that Medicare pays for their care.

It also helps with your outcomes. With everyone speaking the same language, you get a plan and it becomes crystal clear (instead of one physician saying it one way and another physician saying it another way).

Although you may be saying the same thing, it can be interpreted differently because it comes across as being said in different languages. When we have one standardized language in which everyone is speaking, we have much less room for error and much better chances of having quality outcomes.

How does this give Medicare what they want?

- Medicare is asking that you provide clinical validation. √ *CHECK*

- They are asking for you to code your claim appropriately. √ *CHECK*

- And they are asking you to document in a clear and concise manner. √ *CHECK*

By using the Topline Healthcare System and Codeable Language™, your checklist is complete!

Basically, we've taken this complex system and broken it down into an easy to use tool that will help you give Medicare what they want while at the same time, give you more profits and better patient services.

YOUR BEST DEFENSE IS A GOOD OFFENSE

A few years ago, when the government announced that they were going to report data from hospitals and information about you and that it would become public, the physician group of eighteen doctors that I was directly responsible for, averaged a documentation rate of 43%. This means that they weren't hitting anywhere near what Medicare was requiring in order to support a patient's documentation.

I wrote a new note that speaks in Medicare's language and our score went up to 74%. Then, I started educating those physicians on how to document in Codeable Language™ and last year all eighteen of them scored at 93% or above. We were a 550-bed hospital and this had never happened in our facility before. **This program works that well.**

To further ensure that what we document is correct, I became certified as a Clinical Documentation Improvement (CDI) Specialist and I became an RAC coordinator. It was like giving candy to a nerd. Or should I say, giving the right tools to develop a replicable system that will work for healthcare providers across the board so that you can increase your documentation rate and increase your rating publically while increasing your profits.

Understanding the System

For you as a provider, it is as simple as typing in your electronic medical record. When you document within your medical record, we have enabled the system to recognize key phrases as words that may not be acceptable in Medicare language. We have compiled those unacceptable words and have given you a dictionary of words that are acceptable and apply to that particular subject, thus alleviating the need for you to keep all of this in the forefront of your mind.

As time goes on through repetition, you will find yourself documenting in a more appropriate manner and needing to be cued less.

This is a step-by-step program that teaches in real-time as you document, thereby bypassing the need for you to take hours from work to sit in classes. The more you document, the less you will receive prompts, because your appropriately documented note will become second nature, just as it did when you were learning to spell.

Repetition is the Key to Learning

As you work, you are learning. You are learning to increase your profitability, your outcomes, and your patient care. All three of these measurable components increase in quality the more you use the system.

EMPOWER YOURSELF IN FIVE DISTINCTIVE WAYS

ONE:

Patient-Centric Culture

There's a lot of chatter in the medical community currently about "patient first". Being patient-centric is really what Medicare is trying to push providers to do. They state that you need to prove your outcomes, provide the best care possible for the patients and you, as the provider, must lead the way.

If we were talking about football, you would be the quarterback, the one designing the plan. You would then give that information to all of your teammates, from the fullback to the tight end to the defensive end. You have to be able to tell each one of those players what to do while keeping the entire play in your mind.

This is the same as with a provider. You are going to hand this patient off to the nurse. You need to document and tell your team what is going on, keeping that patient ever so much in the forefront of your mind. And you must have faith in the system so that when you hand off the patient, you believe that your team will keep the "patient first."

You must begin to take a good look at outcomes. Look at

the care you are providing as if this were your own mother or father. Would you really want this to be done? Did you think this was necessary?

Many times in my career I have seen things were ordered that I personally didn't feel were necessary. I asked the question of a provider one time, "If this was your mother would you really be doing this test?"

His answer was, "I don't know."

This is one thing you really need to keep in the front of your mind. If this was your mother or father, would you really want this to happen? If this was your child, is this a test or a procedure that you would want done at this juncture of care?

By keeping that in mind, you become patient-centric. You are no longer going through the motions. You are now thinking of this member as your own family and you are going to design care that you feel is the absolute best that can be given.

Patient-centric care is not just a phrase to roll off your tongue. It is a way of life. It is the way of true healthcare. Most likely you went into this line of work because you care about people. You truly want to make them better. Sometimes in the day-to-day grind it's easy to lose sight of that because of the demands from people asking if you have documented or signed off. It can become overwhelming.

But if you stop to think about this being your family, or if this were you, would you do this? You then are not only being patient-centric, but you will then be providing the kind of care that Medicare requires, and more importantly the kind of care that patient is expecting. They trust you with their health and their life. And that is a great honor.

You can begin doing patient-centric care by simply taking five seconds and asking yourself that question each time you are with a patient. This is the foremost philosophy of Topline Healthcare and the culture we fully support building. We can all work together to promote this way of care.

TWO:

Rules, Regulations and Reasons Why

By implementing Codeable Language™, you put yourself in a position to win. This system allows you to document and at the same time be queried so that you don't have to redo work.

Medicare states that anything not documented or that does not support the care is potential fraud. So, as stated previously, if you treat a patient with CHF, don't explain why that patient is there longer than three days, Medicare's guidelines state that the patient's bill is potential fraud.

This program gives you a clear and concise way to document in a very easy, user-friendly manner. As you document, you will be alerted to words that are in question. You will then have to choose from a list of words that are Medicare approved.

You will then be asked if you have the supporting clinical validation. All of these steps fall within the guidelines of CMS so you can document at the top of your game.

As a physician you want to document at the top of your license, and this has never been more important than it is today. Codeable Language™ gives you the most time efficient way to do this.

THREE:

Physician Education and Nuances

With knowledge comes power. Topline Healthcare gives you power by educating physicians as well as coders, thus allowing you to do things in a quick, efficient manner. As you know, time is money, time is important and time is better spent caring for your patients.

Built in the Codeable Language™ program is a secondary and tertiary review system that will allow you to submit a claim that is as clean as possible. This speeds up when your bill gets submitted to Medicare by lessening your accounts receivable days and the amount of times you are queried. This, of course, speeds up the time in which you get paid.

By using this proven method, you will most definitely increase your turnaround time and increase your profitability.

FOUR:

Implementation

Topline Healthcare works with your tech department to implement Codeable Language™ into your electronic medical records. This program also gives a double check to ensure that you are documenting in codeable language.

The application is very simple to use, very simple to install and easily maintained.

One of the great things about this program is that as Medicare makes changes, we are able to send updates, which allows you to start documenting from day one on changes that have been made by Medicare. Unlike a system where you have to manually retrain, this system keeps you updated as Medicare makes those changes. Once they release a blast that talks about a change, that change is implemented immediately in your system.

Instead of taking six months to a year to learn it, you can immediately start documenting because the program, as you use it, teaches you what those changes are and how they affect you. You will receive quick and concise suggestions to ensure your diagnosis meets criteria. This allows you to have continuing education on a daily basis and keeps you on the cutting edge with Medicare.

FIVE:

Data-Gathering and Predictive Modeling

Topline Healthcare is a leader in determining the changes that are coming down the pipe with Medicare. We continually compile information from claims and data and look for trends. We know this is very time consuming and understand that you don't necessarily have time or resources to do this. It requires chart review, looking at data from other regions as well as your own.

It requires you to use your Program for Evaluating Payment Patterns Electronic Report (PEPPER). When Medicare sends out information and the PEPPER report is generated, it tells you where you stand within your region and your state. Most physicians never see this. It's generally used by hospital administrators, your case management department, HIM department and by your CDI department.

Topline Healthcare does this for you. We are a like a coach for you on the sidelines; we see from a distance what the other team is doing and tell you which play to use. We are taking information from all over the country, looking at tracks and trends and then helping you develop a plan based upon your region, your state and what type of work you do. Then we will help you implement that plan within your organization.

This will be supplied to you in a clear, understandable format that keeps you always moving in the right direction so that you not only will win the game, but you can win the championship.

Mark Kimmel, Ph.D.

Chapter 7

How to Get Started

This whole book has been about you developing the mindset of winning at this game of change and putting you on the forefront as a medical leader. Now, it is up to you to position yourself and maintain a high ranking, not only to increase your profits, but also to genuinely provide better patient care and fulfill your mission as a physician.

This is your call to action. With the changes in Medicare rules and regulations, you must act today, because what you are doing today impacts your tomorrow. If what you are documenting now does not meet the standards for CMS, it can become a major financial risk to you as well as a risk to your outcomes.

As you now know, Medicare has changed the rules so that they can go back five years and reclaim money that they feel was given to you inappropriately, or in their view fraudulently due to lack of documentation. Beginning in 2015, Medicare will start taking back reimbursements along this line. That is why your documentation today is as important as your documentation in 2015. Keep this in the forefront of your mind. They will be using the data from

2014 to look for trends. Once they find a trend, they will go back five years, audit you, and take money back.

We are in the forefront of change in medicine. You can protect yourself today by teaming up with us, learning and understanding the changes, and empowering yourself in the five distinctive ways previously discussed.

THE IMPORTANCE OF TAKING ACTION

As a result of the Affordable Care Act, the entire world of medicine is drastically changing, from the way you treat patients to the way you get paid. And when you look at all of the agencies that are now reviewing you as if you are under a microscope (referred to in Chapter 3 and listed in the Index), it is more important now than ever before to take action and protect yourself. Topline Healthcare will design a program specifically for you to help you in the most empowering way.

We are here to educate you on Codeable Language™, to teach you how to use it fully to your advantage. We will help you build a blueprint of success by first, understanding your data, then by implementing programs that help you gather data and track trends. We will offer certification to professionals that will work with you and keep you up to date with the changes in Medicare. By doing so, you will stay ahead of the game, thrive in your career, and genuinely deliver the best care possible.

WHAT YOU NEED TO DO

As you know, the fiscal year for Medicare and for most hospitals starts in October. January 2014 and January 2015 are dates that are coming very quickly. You have to be prepared, and we are here to help.

It is really important for you to get started with an electronic medical record, commonly known as an EMR. It is now virtually impossible to survive without it. If you have not done so already, my guess is that you do not want to do this. I understand. There were many days after the shooting that I did not want to get up and go to work. But I knew I had to in order to survive.

So for you to survive as the provider, you will have to change the way you work, think and feel. That may not be fun or easy. Is it insurmountable? No, it is not. Each step that you take will help you get one step closer, not only to being more profitable, but also to being a better provider and truly serving your patients.

It is time to show your accomplishments and validate all of the good work that you do, and then get fully compensated for doing it. To get started, simply determine in your heart and in your mind that this is something that you can and will do.

Mark Kimmel, Ph.D.

Summary

Author Comments

Many times in my life and in my career, I have been called the fixer. People come to me and ask, "How do I fix this?" I became known as that man who, if you had a problem, would figure out a solution and a way to get it done. It didn't always seem like it was going to work, but I wouldn't give up until did.

What I see for you and what I see for healthcare is a better day coming. Change is always difficult. People fight change because they often dwell in that which is comfortable. We've treated patients the same way in documentation for years. Now we're being asked to change.

When I started in medicine, a profound statement made to me by one of my professors was that medicine changes every five years. And as you know, the art of medicine has certainly changed over the past 20 to 30 years. I remember when we had only a few different antibiotics. Today, we have hundreds of antibiotics at our disposal. That is one of many changes that has improved our industry and given us a better way to treat our patients.

Many times in the past we have felt like we were losing because we couldn't treat our patients to the level we wanted. We didn't have the technology. We didn't have the medicines. Today we now have the technology and the medicines, and we are still growing in that aspect.

The same thing has to be said for our documentation process. It has to grow and evolve. That which has worked for us over the past fifty years no longer works for us today. We live in a digital age that requires us to be faster and far more efficient. It requires us to use everything we have at our disposal to treat patients better. I believe that we have started this process, we will complete this process, and we will come out on the other side of this together much stronger and much, much better.

Patient-centric care is not only asking if you would do this for your family, it is also asking yourself if, God forbid, you dropped dead tomorrow, could your colleague come in and know what you know about this patient. If I should fall and break my leg and I was supposed to go in and see Mrs. Jones, I know that my colleague could come in and take care of this patient just like I can because we are speaking the same language. We see the same thing. We then move together as one, solid component instead of three or four working around each other. We move together truly as a united team.

We have come together, created this magnificently unstoppable team, and are forging ahead to create a better future for everyone. I truly appreciate you being this on journey with us and admire your courage.

I know often times this kind of book can be, shall I say, very dry. But I thank you for taking the time to read it anyway and for positively looking into your future. I thank you for understanding that this is really about you, this is about your patients, and this is about believing in your success.

Our success comes when you are successful. We appreciate that you have taken the time to go through the articles and understand our concepts. Above all, we are most grateful that you care enough about your patients to spend the time and energy to stay ahead of the game. Because at the end of the day it is not only about us, but it's about the people we care for and the strength of the care we give.

Very truly yours,

Mark Kimmel, Ph.D.

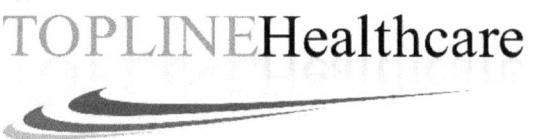

www.toplinehealthcare.com

Index

List of Agencies and Other Acronyms

LIST OF AGENCIES
(From Chapter 3)

CERT - Comprehensive Error Rate Testing: Measures improper payments in the Medicare fee-for-service (FFS) program and to monitor the accuracy with which Medicare claims are billed and paid. *(15, 47)*

CMS - Centers for Medicare & Medicaid Services: The Federal agency, of the Department of Health and Human Services that, among other things, is responsible for administering Medicare and Medicaid. *(6, 14, 24, 29, 30, 42, 43, 45, 76 — 82, 83, 87, 89, 96)*

DOJ - Department of Justice: Promotes and establish justice and the appearance of justice by vigorously and fairly representing the United States and its citizens in all matters, civil or criminal, within their jurisdiction. *(24, 47)*

HCC - Hierarchical Condition Categories: The goal of the CMS HCC Medicare risk adjustment is to pay Medicare Advantage (MA) and Prescription Drug Plans (PDPs) accurately and fairly by adjusting payment for enrollees based on demographics and health status. *(9, 82)*

HEAT - Health Care Fraud Prevention and Enforcement Action Team: Prevents waste, fraud, and abuse in the Medicare and Medicaid programs and crack down on the people and organizations abusing the system. *(47)*

IPA - Independent Practice Association: An association of independent physicians (or other organization that contracts with independent physicians) and provides services to managed care organizations on a negotiated per capita rate, flat retainer fee, or negotiated fee-for-service basis. *(10, 36, 41)*

IPIA – Improper Payments Information Act: Purpose is to annually review programs they administer and identify those that may be susceptible to significant improper payments, to estimate the amount of improper payments, to submit those estimates to Congress, and to submit a report on actions the agency is taking to reduce the improper payments. *(47)*

MIC - Medicaid Integrity Contractors: Provide anti-fraud education to Medicaid providers and to identify overpayments by conducting post-payment audits of Medicaid claims. (47)

MIP - Medicaid Integrity Program: Prevents and reduces provider fraud, waste, and abuse in the $300 billion per year Medicaid program. *(47)*

MMA - Medicare Administrative Contractor: Makes Medicare contract awards more competitive and contracts more efficient. *(47)*

OIG - Office of Inspector General: Protects the integrity of Department of Health & Human Services (HHS) programs as well as the health and welfare of program beneficiaries. *(24, 46, 48)*

PERM- Payment Error Rate Measurement: Measures improper payments in Medicaid and CHIP and produces error rates for each program. The error rates are based upon fee-for-service (FFS), managed care, and eligibility components of Medicaid and CHIP in the fiscal year under review. *(48)*

PSC - Program Safeguard Contractors: The Health Insurance Portability and Accountability Act (HIPAA) authorized the Centers for Medicare & Medicaid Services () to contract with entities known as Program Safeguard Contractors to conduct Medicare program integrity activities such as conducting post-payment audits of providers to ensure that claims have been appropriately billed. *(48)*

RAC - Recovery Audit Contractor: Identify and correct Medicare improper payments through the efficient detection and collection of overpayments made on claims of healthcare services provided to Medicare beneficiaries, and the identification of underpayments to providers so that the CMS can implement actions that will prevent future improper payments in all 50 states. *(1, 8, 10, 14—15, 23-25, 30—33, 47—48, 53, 56—57, 60—61, 72, 75—78, 93)*

ZPIC - Zone Program Integrity Contractor: Combats fraud, waste, and abuse in the Medicare program. ZPICs replaced Program Safeguard Contractors (PSC), which had been established by the Health Insurance Portability and Accountability Act of 1996. *(24, 48)*

OTHER ACRONYMS

ALJ - Administrative Law Judge *(30, 60—61)*

CC - Comorbidities *(67)*

CDI - Clinical Documentation Improvement *(42, 53, 69, 85, 93, 99)*

CHF - Congestive Heart Failure *(20, 50, 96)*

CLS - Codeable Language Specialist *(85)*

DHHS - Department of Health and Human Services *(23)*

DRG - Diagnosis Related Group *(73,81)*

GERD - Gastro esophageal reflux disease *(20, 41, 58, 77)*

EMR - Electronic Medical Record *(43, 45, 50, 69, 79, 103)*

HIM - Health Information Management *(22, 23, 99)*

HIPAA - Health Insurance Portability and Accountability Act *(37, 39)*

HITECH - Health Information Technology for Economic and Clinical Health Act *(35)*

HPMP - Hospital Payment Monitoring Program *(15)*

ICD-9, ICD-10 - International Statistical Classifications of Diseases current codes in use. *(1,14–16, 21, 32, 78)*

JCAHO - Joint Commission on Accreditation of Healthcare Organizations *(42–43, 45, 72)*

MCC - Major Comorbidities *(67)*

PEPPER - Program for Evaluating Payment Patterns Electronic Report *(98)*

QIO - Quality Improvement Organization *(15)*

About the Author

Mark Kimmel, Ph.D.

A California Christian University graduate with a PhD in both Education and Theology, Mark Kimmel has been in the medical field for over 20 years, from working in hospitals caring for others, leading and creating programs, to doing medical missionary work throughout the world.

He is known for his skills in leadership, clinical knowledge and understanding of workflows. He became a nurse working in ICU, Trauma, and Case Management. While working with Care Management at one of the nation's top hospitals in Southern California, Mark was instrumental in the development of computer processes that lead to the hospital receiving the Franklin Award of Distinction which is a competitive, annual award sponsored by the American Case Management Association (ACMA), and The Joint Commission that recognizes distinctive organizational Case Management performance.

Mark is the creator of Codeable Language™ and co-founder of Topline Healthcare, a computer software system and training program that assists hospitals and healthcare providers with clinical documentation, which has proven to help save time and money while increasing profitability and quality of care.

In addition to helping several local charities and non-profits over the years, Mark has served with Operation Blessing International Relief and Development Corporation to provide food globally to those in need.

Mark's life long passion for working with medical missions, taking care of others and innovating the healthcare industry continues to this day.